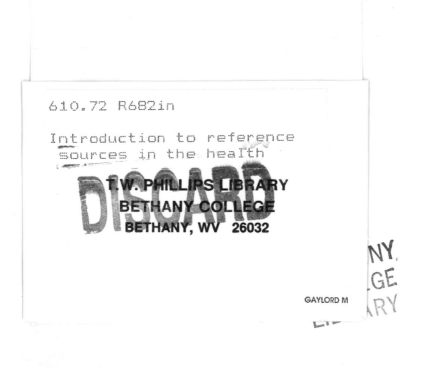

Introduction to
Reference Sources
in the
Health Sciences

LIST OF AUTHORS

JO ANNE BOORKMAN
Assistant Director for Public Services
Health Sciences Library
University of North Carolina at Chapel Hill
Chapel Hill, NC

SANDRA COLVILLE-STEWART
Head, History & Special Collections Division
Biomedical Library
University of California at Los Angeles
Los Angeles, CA

REBECCA W. DAVIDSON
Coordinator of Automated Reference Services
Health Sciences Library
University of North Carolina at Chapel Hill
Chapel Hill, NC

RICHARD HINSON
Reference Librarian
Health Sciences Library
University of North Carolina at Chapel Hill
Chapel Hill, NC

J. MICHAEL HOMAN
Head, Information Services
Corporate Technical Library
The Upjohn Company
Kalamazoo, MI

JULIE KUENZEL KWAN
Head, Reference Department
Biomedical Library
University of California at Los Angeles
Los Angeles, CA

TAYLOR PUTNEY
Coordinator of Public Services
Health Sciences Library
Wright State University
Dayton, OH

FRED W. ROPER
Assistant Dean and Associate Professor
School of Library Science
University of North Carolina at Chapel Hill
Chapel Hill, NC

Introduction to Reference Sources in the Health Sciences

by
FRED W. ROPER
and
JO ANNE BOORKMAN

Medical Library Association, Inc.

Chicago, Illinois

National Library of Medicine Cataloging in Publication

Roper, Fred Wilburn
Introduction to reference sources in the health sciences
by Fred Roper and Jo Anne Boorkman.—Chicago
Medical Library Assn., 1980.

1. Bibliography of Medicine   2. Information Services–U.S.
I. Boorkman, Jo Anne.   II. Medical Library Association.   III. Title.

04NLM:ZWB 100 R784i

ISBN 0-912176-08-3

This book
is for my parents,
RUTH and CHARLES BOORKMAN (JAB)
and for my Mother,
MARY ALICE JONES,
and the memory of my Stepfather,
GEORGE JONES (FWR)

CONTENTS

PREFACE

The purpose of *Introduction to Reference Sources in the Health Sciences* is to discuss various types of bibliographic and informational sources and their use in reference work in the health sciences. Although the book is written with the library school student in mind, practicing librarians and health science library users should also find the book to be of value.

Since it is difficult to cover the whole field of the health sciences in depth, the work is selective, giving the tools that librarians may use on a daily basis in reference work in the health sciences—those tools that may be considered foundation or basic works. Some of the major specialized tools have been included, but there is no attempt to go into subject specialization in great detail. Emphasis is placed on United States publications and libraries.

The introduction to the reference collection in the opening section is intended as a basis for the discussion of the different categories of reference materials that follows. Since the fourth edition of the *Handbook of Medical Library Practice* is currently in preparation, no attempt has been made to present an extensive discussion of reference services in this book.

The major portions of the book present the different types of bibliographic and informational sources. Each chapter contains a discussion of the general characteristics of the type being considered, followed by examples of the most important tools in the area. Emphasis is put on the use of materials and, where appropriate, a comparison with similar materials is included. If available, suggested additional readings are included for each topic. For the most part, the readings are limited to materials published after 1970.

Since no consensus exists as to what constitutes "basic works," the materials here represent the authors' candidates for such a list. In many instances other, equally appropriate examples could have been selected. For certain groups of sources, e.g., technical report literature, materials that are considerably broader in scope than the health science field alone have been included to help the reader toward a clear understanding of the use of these sources in reference work in the health sciences.

PART I

The Reference Collection

CHAPTER 1

Organization and Management
of the
Reference Collection

JO ANNE BOORKMAN

What exactly is a reference collection? How does it differ from other parts of the library's collection? What characterizes the materials in the reference collection? How are they selected, organized, and maintained?

Reference collections evolve and develop from the nature of reference work. In addition to carrying out literature searches, reference librarians are most frequently called on for assistance in answering factual and bibliographic questions. The tools most frequently used to answer these types of questions make up the reference collection; materials in this collection are consulted for specific and immediate information instead of being read from beginning to end. To assure that these materials are available for immediate and short-term use, the reference collection is separated from the circulating collections of the library, placed in an easily accessible library service area, and made noncirculating. It should be noted that medical reference tools frequently require the assistance of a trained medical librarian for effective use.

This book introduces a number of works considered to be desirable tools in a health sciences library's reference collection. All are appropriate, if not essential, for a large library. Smaller libraries will need to be selective in acquiring the most appropriate tools for their collections.

Little has been written on the nature of the reference collection and of the policies for developing and maintaining it. Selection policies,[1,2] while generally discussing the collection as a whole, usually define four levels of coverage for subject areas: comprehensive/exhaustive, research, reference, and skeletal. These can be described as follows:

1. *Exhaustive*. For a subject collected on the exhaustive level, the library will obtain copies of all editions of all books, journals, pamphlets, reports, and so on, dealing with the subject and published at any time in any language. All manuscript materials relating to this subject will also be acquired.

2. *Research*. For a subject collected on the research level, the library will obtain the current or best edition of the books, journals, pamphlets, reports, and documents in the commonly used languages that are necessary to permit independent research on a doctoral level.

3. *Reference*. For a subject collected on the reference level, the library will obtain a current dictionary, a current encyclopedia, the latest or best editions of several texts, a comprehensive bibliography, one or more journals, an indexing or abstracting journal, and one or more histories.

4. *Skeletal*. For a subject collected on the skeletal level, the library will obtain a current dictionary, the latest or best edition of one or two texts, and a history.[3]

Regardless of the level at which the material is collected, the subject should be represented in both the reference *and* general collections of the library. Therefore, simply defining a level of coverage does not adequately answer the question, "Which materials should comprise a reference collection?"

A reference collection policy should be developed as a document parallel to the overall collection development policy of the library. It should be defined not only in relation to the research and educational goals of the particular institution but also in relation to the types of materials most often used in the reference situation.

Consideration should also be given to the format of materials, both print and nonprint, in the reference collection. Specifically, will tools available only in microform be acceptable? Which types of tools will be considered for purchase in print form? In microform? In which other formats?

Online sources of both bibliographic information and factual data can be considered to be a part of the reference collection and should be included as a possible format for reference tools in the collection policy statement. It could be argued that online sources form a separate reference service; however, they are considered here as an additional format for some of the most heavily used reference tools: indexes, abstracts, and drug/chemical sources.

A third area to consider is duplication of materials. Some tools, such as heavily used textbooks, should be considered for both the circulating and reference collections. Likewise, duplicate copies of heavily used reference books, e.g., medical dictionaries or the *Physicians' Desk Reference (PDR)*, may be needed at the reference desk and in the reference office in addition to the reference collection.

In the following example of a reference collection policy outline, consideration of formats and multiple copies have been listed separately for illustrative purposes. They could be incorporated into part III under each specific category following the scope-of-coverage statement.

Outline for a Reference Collection Policy[1,4]

  I. Introduction
     A. History of the policy
        1. Date of the original formulation
        2. Authority establishing the policy
     B. Present revision of the policy with the date of approval
 II. Purpose
     A. General scope statement for the reference collection
     B. Definition of reference coverage by subject
        in relation to the overall collection policy
        of the library
III. Categories of reference materials
     A. Information on persons, organizations, or institutions
        1. Directories of persons—biographical directories
        2. Directories of organizations
        3. Telephone directories
     B. Factual data
        1. Dictionaries
           (a) General English-language
           (b) Subject
           (c) Foreign-language
        2. Encyclopedias
        3. Handbooks
        4. Drug sources
        5. Statistical sources
        6. Legislation, regulations
           (a) Federal
           (b) State
           (c) Local

      7. Catalogs
        (*a*) Educational institutions
        (*b*) Commercial products, including laboratory
           and audiovisual equipment and supplies
      8. Manuals and guides
        (*a*) Writing and style manuals
        (*b*) Online search manuals
      9. Indexes, abstracts, and bibliographies
     10. Lists of meetings
   C. Union lists and catalogs
      1. Book catalogs
      2. Serial sources
        (*a*) Union lists
        (*b*) Abbreviations lists, lists of journals
           indexed/abstracted (included by indexing
           and abstract services)
      3. Audiovisual software sources
        (*a*) Catalogs from producers
        (*b*) Union lists
      4. Translation sources
   D. Textbooks and histories
   E. Ephemeral and pamphlet materials
 IV. Format
   A. Print
   B. Nonprint
      1. Microforms
      2. Online data bases
 V. Multiple copies
   A. Serials, e.g., *Index Medicus*
      1. Determination of need
      2. Locations: reference, reference office,
        journal stacks, etc.
   B. Books, e.g., medical dictionary, *PDR*, etc.
      1. Determination of need
      2. Locations: reference stacks, reference desk,
        reference office, reading room(s), etc.
   C. Online search tools
      1. Determination of need
      2. Locations: reference office, terminal location(s),
        reference desk, etc.

The reference collection policy should not be considered an academic exercise. It is a concrete means by which a collection can be measured and developed. This outline provides a framework for developing a policy, but a policy, like a collection, must be reviewed regularly to determine if it fulfills the goals of maintaining a vital reference collection. The policy should be considered a creative tool.

Along with the collection development policy for reference, there should be a sensible weeding/retention policy. Many reference tools come out in new editions at regular intervals—annually or biennially, for example. It would be impossible to maintain a usable reference collection if all these editions were kept in the reference collection. Unlike weeding for the general collection, in which materials are discarded or offered on exchange to other libraries, a reference weeding policy has the option of retiring earlier editions of reference tools to the general circulating collection. Of course, duplicate copies could be withdrawn; two copies of the 1979 *AHA Guide to the Health Care Field* in the circulating collection would not be sensible when there are two copies of the current edition in the reference collection. One copy is sufficient for comparative or historical purposes.

In some instances, however, it is useful to keep more than one edition of a tool in the reference collection. For example, the 1977 edition of the *Canadian Medical Directory* lists Canadian hospitals and nursing homes and their addresses. That section was omitted in subsequent editions. It is, therefore, advisable not to remove the earlier edition from the reference collection unless there is a separate source, such as the *Canadian Hospital Directory*, for this hospital information.

A reference collection weeding policy could be outlined as follows:

Reference Weeding Policy Outline
  I. Introduction
     A. History of the policy
       1. Date of original formulation
       2. Authority establishing the policy
     B. Present revision of the policy with date of approval
 II. Purpose
III. Retention
     (To be coordinated with the overall collection development
     policy for areas in which exhaustive collections or
     archival material would always be kept.)

A. Latest edition only kept in library on reference (primary materials that supersede themselves)
  1. Online manuals
  2. Individual libraries' holdings lists
  3. Pamphlets
  4. Catalogs (college, audiovisual producers, equipment, etc.)
B. Latest edition on reference, earlier editions in the circulating collection
  1. Any category A materials found to be unique and worth retaining in the collection for historical or research purposes
  2. Dictionaries
  3. Directories
  4. Handbooks
  5. Drug sources
  6. Textbooks
  7. Encyclopedias
  8. Writing and style manuals
  9. Book catalogs
C. Earlier editions kept on reference as their usefulness to reference and available space permit
  1. Any category B materials containing unique information found useful to reference
  2. Indexes and abstracting services
  3. Bibliographies
  4. Statistical sources
  5. Union lists and serials sources
  6. Translation sources
  7. Lists of meetings

A separate outline for a weeding policy has been given; however, retention information could logically be incorporated into the reference collection policy for each category of reference tool.

Access to the tools in the reference collection is generally through the public catalog, with a stamped note or plastic overlay on the card indicating that an item is in the reference collection, or with "also in reference" on the catalog card for items that are in the general collection and duplicated in reference. Larger libraries may want to have a separate reference catalog or reference shelflist for access to the reference collection alone. However, in libraries where the reference collection is small, items in the general collection may be used more frequently than in large libraries to answer patrons' questions; in this case access to all items, including reference materials, through a single public catalog would be preferable. The availability of an online interactive catalog, where the patron can query the catalog and get a response, may be a possibility at larger libraries in the not-too-distant future. This may provide yet another means of access to the reference collection.

How should the reference collection be organized? There are varying schools of thought on this subject. A reference collection consists of both monographic and serial publications. The monographic collection will probably be classified by means of the National Library of Medicine's classification system or some other scheme. The serial collection may or may not be classified; many libraries prefer to arrange their serials alphabetically. Some additional questions may arise concerning serials in the reference collection: Are reference serials to be classified or arranged alphabetically? Which items are considered serials in reference? Just the indexes and abstracts, or all serial publications?

If an entirely classified arrangement is chosen, the collection is usually shelved by classified (subject) arrangement regardless of the type or format of the material. An exception is often made for indexes and abstracts, which are arranged on index tables for ease of use.

A modification of the classified arrangement can also be used in which the monographic collection is classified and arranged by call number, but the serial publications are not classified and are arranged alphabetically. These are primarily indexes and abstracts, but can also include other serial publications (like World Meetings, Unlisted Drugs, and Vital and Health Statistics) usually found in a reference collection. In practice, some libraries classify reference serials; others leave them alphabetically arranged; and others group them chronologically, as is frequently done with the medical indexes, Index Medicus and its predecessors. One real problem with the alphabetically arranged serials collection arises when the title of a work changes, separating consecutive volumes of the work.

The monographic reference collection, while classified, may not always be arranged strictly by call number. Some reference departments prefer an arrangement by form categories[5,6] (see example following) in which all dictionaries, directories, handbooks, etc., are shelved together. These categories are not arranged just by form, however. Some provide subject grouping like "drug lists," which includes handbooks, dictionaries, manuals, etc., on the subject. Other libraries have a combination of a classified arrangement with a form arrangement for heavily used items like dictionaries, directories, textbooks, and college catalogs. When such arrangements are used, proper labeling of the public catalog and of the reference collection is essential to guide the user to the location of the material in the reference area.

Reference Categories

1. Dictionaries (medical and other subjects; English and foreign; also includes nomenclature, terminology, and quotation lists)
2. Manuals and guides (style manuals, writing guides, programmed texts on medical terminology, legal and ethical manuals)
3. Almanacs and statistical compilations (includes all reference materials on statistics)
4. Subject handbooks (data books such as *Handbook of Chemistry and Physics, Biology Data Handbook, Handbook of Clinical Laboratory Data*)
5. Drug lists (all reference materials on drugs, including manuals, dictionaries, and handbooks)
6. Biographical directories (includes all reference materials listing people)
7. Directories (includes listings of institutions, organizations, scholarships, educational programs, agencies)
8. Geographical atlases (includes geographical material such as *Webster's Atlas and Zip Code Directory, Hotel and Motel Red Book*)
9. Encyclopedias and encyclopedic works (such as *Encyclopaedia Britannica, Handbook of Experimental Pharmacology, Practice of Medicine*)
10. Library information (includes directories, handbooks, and manuals in the field of library science)
11. Bibliographies and histories (includes selected bibliographies in the health sciences, history of medicine, and nonprint media)
12. Serials information (includes union catalogs, abbreviation lists, directories of periodicals such as *Ulrich's International Periodicals Directory*)

13. Book catalogs (includes listings of books such as *Books in Print, National Library of Medicine Current Catalog, Cumulative Book Index*)
14. Lists of meetings and translations (such as *Technical Translations Index, World Meetings U.S. and Canada, Annual International Congress Calendar*)

Whatever arrangement is chosen, consideration must be made for ease of use by the library user as well as the reference librarian. Jeuell, in presenting an arrangement by categories, argues that arrangement by form increases the retrievability of information from the collection, since patrons frequently want a *type* of information, e.g., biographical, but may not know the subject area in which to look. A classified arrangement would require looking for biographies in several subject areas. She concludes:

> Form arrangement results in efficient use of the monographic collection by making it more retrievable, in terms of the patron's information needs, than a straight call number arrangement. Arrangement by form takes into account that some vital information might be missing from a reference question, and that many patrons use a monographic reference collection by browsing through a group of similar books such as biographical directories, rather than looking for a subject or for a specific title in the card catalog.[5]

On the other hand, arrangement by form can lead to arbitrary placement of books in a category. Some items are neither strictly handbooks, statistical sources, nor directories. In which category should they be placed? How efficiently is the patron then served? Subject arrangement (classified) *does* scatter similar forms of publications; however, it increases "browsability" within a field of interest—ophthalmology, hospitals, nursing, etc.

Of course, there are some times when form arrangement would have its advantages and other times when subject arrangement would be more advantageous. The arrangement chosen will depend on how the reference staff uses the collection and how they perceive the majority of patrons' use of the collection—by form or by subject.

The physical arrangement of the collection will also depend to a great extent on the space available. Whether the "ideal" arrangement is considered to be by form categories, classified, or a combination of classified and alphabetic, the actual arrangement may be determined by where the collection can be housed. There may not be enough room for all the indexes and abstracts to fit on index tables. Which ones, then, should be arranged on the tables? In what order? Obviously, *Index Medicus* should be there, but volumes for how many years should be kept at this access point?

As for the monographic reference collection and other reference serials, are they near the reference desk? If not, should the collection be split to provide quick access to the most frequently used tools? Or should the collection have duplicate copies of heavily used items, one set for the reference stacks and one for the reference desk? Is there space available at the desk? Will space constraints determine the use of form arrangement versus classified subject arrangement?

If space is at a premium, should microform (film or fiche) be considered as the primary format for some tools? If so, which ones? *Chemical Abstracts?* Telephone books? Medical school and college catalogs? How are these to be arranged in relation to the other tools in the collection? Is there space for microform readers in the reference area? How many are needed?

These are just a few of the questions that must be considered in deciding how to arrange a reference collection. There is no perfect answer—each library has a collection unique in size and content, based on the usage and reference demands of its clientele. How the collection is arranged should be determined by these usage and reference patterns to maximize efficient use of the collection within the space constraints of the building. Easy, logical access to the collection by the users and staff should be the goal for a collection's organization and physical arrangement.

Maintaining the collection is an ongoing process. Current addresses, telephone numbers, statistical data, etc., are often the information sought from a reference tool. To answer such questions, it is important to have the latest available edition of a tool in the collection. There are several ways to keep current: (1) publishers' announcements, (2) acquisitions lists of other health sciences libraries, and (3) online cataloging files.

In a large library, the reference librarian(s) working with the acquisitions and collections development staff can be alerted to forthcoming editions of reference tools already in the collection as well as newly published tools to consider adding to the collection. Publishers frequently send out notices announcing these new titles and editions.

When new reference tools are selected, the guidelines from the reference collection policy should be followed. Is the tool going to provide new information? Does it duplicate information available in other tools? If so, is the information in a more easily retrievable format, making this new tool a desirable acquisition? Often this information is not discernible from a publisher's announcement. It may then be advisable to wait to purchase the item until a review is published in a library journal like the *Bulletin of the Medical Library Association* or until the item appears on the acquisitions list of another health sciences library. In the latter case, that library can be contacted for an opinion; or it can be assumed that because that library purchased it, the item is acceptable, although making this assumption has its pitfalls unless the library's reference selection policy is known. Another source for reviews of new tools is in the various regional medical library newsletters. These are aimed at smaller and hospital libraries and can provide guides in selecting for such collections.

Using the cataloging data bases as aids in selection also can be helpful. Both the National Library of Medicine's CATLINE (*CAT* alog on *LINE*) file and the OCLC, Inc., data base can be used in ascertaining the latest edition of a particular work; CATLINE is particularly useful in identifying new material in a subject field, while SERLINE (*SER* ials on *LINE*) can provide similar information for periodicals.

Materials in some areas are particularly difficult to keep current. Directories of specialized societies are often published once and then abandoned or are published only sporadically. Statistical sources can also be a problem. A study may be done once and then never updated. For these and other difficult areas, a systematic and regular inventory of the reference collection is necessary. By this means one can identify those areas that need to be updated and strengthened with new editions of existing tools or with tools that have previously been overlooked but could be useful in the collection. There is always a reference question for which there may be a better source than the ones available in the collection. Keeping an eye out for that source helps maintain a current and vital reference collection.

The purpose of this chapter has not been to provide answers. It is intended to present the issues relating to the way a reference collection is developed, organized, and maintained. There are many factors to consider. The questions raised here will, it is hoped, lead to thoughtful consideration of how best to organize a new collection, or an existing one, or even to assess how an existing collection came to be the way it is. The important question is: How can the collection best serve the user?

REFERENCES

[1] Beatty, W. K. Technical Processes: Part 1. Selection, Acquisition and Weeding. In: Annan, Gertrude L. and Felter, Jacqueline W., eds., *Handbook of Medical Library Practice*. 3rd ed. Chicago, IL, Medical Library Association, 1970. pp. 71–92.

[2] National Library of Medicine. Technical Services Division. *Scope and Coverage Manual of the National Library of Medicine*. Bethesda, MD, National Library of Medicine, May, 1977.

[3] Beatty, W. K., *op. cit.*, p. 73.

[4] Houston Academy of Medicine—Texas Medical Center Library. *Collection Development Policy*. Apr., 1978 (unpublished manuscript).

[5] Jeuell, C. A., The Reorganization of a Monographic Reference Collection. *Bull. Med. Lib. Assoc.* 64: 293–298, Jul., 1976.

[6] Truelson, S. C., Jr. The Totally Organized Reference Collection. *Bull. Med. Lib. Assoc.* 50: 184–187, Apr., 1962.

PART II

Bibliographic Sources

CHAPTER 2

Bibliographic Sources
for
Monographs

FRED W. ROPER

Although the monograph is no longer the primary means of printed communication in the health sciences, it remains an important component of all library collections, and materials for bibliographic control of monographs are an integral part of any reference collection.

The basic purposes of these materials are verification, location, and selection.[1]

The process of *verification* involves establishment for each item of the needed bibliographic elements, such as author, title, place of publication, and collation. In seeking to verify various bibliographic elements related to one title, it may be necessary to consult several sources. The most useful sources are generally those that are comprehensive in scope.

Location refers to the actual library in which a title may be found or the source from which it may be purchased. Printed library catalogs and union catalogs are the primary tools for determining library holdings. Trade bibliographies indicating which titles, regardless of age, are still offered for sale by publishers are used to determine availability for purchase.

Since collection development is such an important part of the librarian's work, the *selection* function presupposes bibliographies that indicate materials available in a given subject area, by a particular author, or in a given format. Often bibliographies will provide an evaluation of an item's worth or an indication of its content in the form of an annotation.

Bibliographies in the health sciences field may perform more than one of these three functions and are likely to contain entries for more than one type of material: monographs, periodicals, government documents, and so on.

CURRENT SOURCES

Current coverage of medical monographs is primarily carried out by the National Library of Medicine (NLM) using the CATLINE data base and its printed products.

2.1 CATLINE (*CAT* alog on *LINE*). Bethesda, MD, National Library of Medicine.

2.2 *National Library of Medicine Current Catalog*. Bethesda, MD, National Library of Medicine. 1966– . Quarterly; annual and five-year cumulations.

2.3 *National Library of Medicine Current Catalog Proof Sheets*. Chicago, IL, Medical Library Association. Weekly.

The CATLINE data base, an online system from NLM, contains more than 200,000 citations cataloging information for all serials and monographs cataloged or recataloged by NLM since 1965, as well as cataloging information supplied by several participating libraries. It represents the most up-to-date compilation of cataloging information for materials in the health sciences and is the data base from which the major printed cataloging products are derived.

The most significant of these printed tools is the *National Library of Medicine Current Catalog*, which is published quarterly with annual and five-year cumulations. It succeeds earlier NLM catalogs, which had been printed as supplements to the Library of Congress's catalogs from 1948 to 1965.

The quarterly issues contain citations to items that were cataloged during the three-month period covered by that issue, except for those items published before 1801. Both monographs and serials are included, with a separate subject and main entry section for each type of material. The full entry is found only under the main entry, with added entries taking the form of cross-references to the main entry. Each citation includes standard bibliographic information plus (when available) Library of Congress card number, the price in United States currency, and the International Standard Book Number (ISBN) or International Standard Serial Number (ISSN).

The NLM *Classification Scheme* (4th edition, 1978), is generally used, although titles in peripheral fields are classified according to the Library of Congress (LC) classification schedules with no modification. Subject headings are from *Medical Subject Headings (MeSH) Annotated Alphabetic List*, NLM's subject heading list, which is used in the preparation of the other NLM bibliographies and indexes. Individuals and corporate bodies appearing as subjects are listed in the main entry sections ("name" sections) rather than in the "subject" sections. Of particular importance to reference libraries is the use of the heading "Reference Books, Medical." Since January 1973, this descriptor has been employed to bring together in the subject section for monographs a selection of recently cataloged reference books.

After each weekly update to the CATLINE data base, the *Current Catalog Proof Sheets*, distributed by the Medical Library Association, are photocomposed. The *Proof Sheets* contain only English-language citations from the current three years of the data base. This publication represents the most timely printed version of NLM cataloging. Because of its currency, it is useful in the selection and acquisitions processes.

Since medical monographs are also included in the *National Union Catalog* and other general bibliographic tools, such as *Cumulative Book Index*, *Weekly Record*, and *American Book Publishing Record*, these tools, too, are useful in the verification and location of medical monographs.

2.4 *National Union Catalog: A Cumulative Author List.* Washington, DC, Library of Congress, Card Division. 1956– . Nine monthly issues; three quarterly cumulations.

2.5 *Cumulative Book Index.* New York, NY, H. W. Wilson. 1898– . Monthly; three-month, annual, and five-year cumulations.

2.6 *American Book Publishing Record.* New York, NY, Bowker. 1961– . Monthly; annual cumulation.

2.7 *Weekly Record.* New York, NY, Bowker. 1974– . Weekly.

The *National Union Catalog (NUC)* provides a listing of materials currently cataloged by LC, regardless of imprint date, and by participating libraries throughout the United States and Canada, for imprints 1956 and later if the material has not previously been cataloged by LC. Because of the extremely large number of items included in *NUC*, it represents a vast bibliographic resource for a large part of the world's output of monographs and other types of material.

The series of catalogs published by NLM from 1948 to 1965 served as supplements to the LC catalogs in the field of medicine and related subjects. With the inauguration of the *Current Catalog* in 1966, however, the NLM catalog was no longer a supplement to the LC catalogs. Present catalog entries from NLM with an imprint date of 1956 or later are included in the *NUC*, as are entries for works in medicine acquired and cataloged by the Library of Congress and by the other participating libraries.

The *NUC* is issued on a monthly basis with three quarterly cumulations; these are followed by annual and five-year cumulations. For an extensive discussion of the history, development, and scope of the *National Union Catalog*, the reader is referred to the "Foreword" that appears in each issue.

Entries may appear in the *NUC* only if a participating library has acquired and cataloged an item; thus *NUC* serves not only as a verification source but also as a location source.

The *Cumulative Book Index* and the *American Book Publishing Record* represent two ongoing bibliographic sources that attempt to provide bibliographic information about English-language publications in all subject areas. As such, they are important to the librarian in the health sciences. Their primary purpose is to list books that can be purchased from publishers (mostly American). Each will provide enough information to order an item. Over a period of time, their cumulations provide a record of what has been published in the United States or in the English language elsewhere.

The *Weekly Record* and its companion work, the *American Book Publishing Record*, provide a weekly and monthly listing of new books being published in the United States only. The scope of the *Cumulative Book Index* is broader than that of the *Weekly Record* and the *American Book Publishing Record*: its goal is to provide an international bibliography of books in the English language.

2.8 *Books in Print.* New York, NY, Bowker. 1948– . Annual. *Books in Print Supplement.* New York, NY, Bowker. 1973– . Annual.

2.9 *Medical Books and Serials in Print.* New York, NY, Bowker. 1978– . Annual.

2.10 Kyed, James M., and Matarazzo, James M. *Scientific, Engineering, and Medical Societies Publications in Print, 1978–1979.* New York, NY, Bowker, 1979.

A recurring question in bibliographic work has to do with the availability for purchase of a particular item. Is it still in print and for sale? A group of publications from the R. R. Bowker Company will be of assistance with this type of question.

Books in Print (BIP) provides an author and title approach to approximately 500,000 books, in all subject areas, which are still in print. Each entry includes the source from which the book can be purchased and how much it costs, along with other bibliographic elements, such as year of publication, ISBN, and LC card number. The addresses of those publishers included in *BIP* are listed in a special section. Most of the titles listed in *BIP* can be found in the subject companion, *Subject Guide to Books in Print,* which uses LC headings.

These two titles are prepared from a computer data base maintained by the Bowker Company to compile their various "in-print" publications. Another title produced from this data base of direct interest to the health sciences is *Medical Books and Serials in Print.* Dealing exclusively with the health sciences, its stated objective is

> to produce as comprehensive a guide as possible to literature in health and biomedical sciences. The indexes to books list titles which are in-print and have been or will be published or exclusively distributed in the United States. . . . The coverage of the serial indexes is international and contains selected titles of periodicals issued more frequently than once a year and usually published at regular intervals, and/or irregular serials and annuals provided in the last issue date was not earlier than 1968.

This work is likely to be of greatest value to the smaller library that cannot afford to have an extensive collection of bibliographic tools.

Another Bowker publication that includes medical materials is *Scientific, Engineering, and Medical Societies Publications in Print 1978– 1979,* which brings together in one source information about the societies and their publishing programs, including monographs, serials, and a wide variety of nonbook materials. A wide range of audience levels is represented in the work, which indicates the availability of all the materials listed.

RETROSPECTIVE SOURCES

From the time of the development of the printing press in the fifteenth century until the nineteenth century, the printed book was the primary source for information. By the mid-nineteenth century, the periodical had so increased in use and number that it replaced the book in importance. Increasingly larger amounts of materials were being printed, and the sheer bulk of the literature made it no longer possible to be aware of everything being published.

Although bibliographies of medical materials had been publi: ˑd prior to the mid-nineteenth century, they had not attempted to be ɩ inclusive and were therefore selective in their coverage. For the mosɩ part they were concerned with books, although in many the contents of periodicals were included as well. In addition to those bibliographies that were concerned solely or primarily with medical materials, the general bibliographic tools of the early periods need to be consulted, since many medical items will be included in them. For a detailed account of early bibliographic coverage of medical materials, the reader should consult *The Development of Medical Bibliography* by Estelle Brodman.[2]

The "father of medical bibliography" was John Shaw Billings. As librarian of the Surgeon-General's Library, the forerunner of NLM, Billings was responsible for publication of the *Index-Catalogue of the Library of the Surgeon-General's Office* and for the original *Index Medicus*. These two publications marked the beginning of a consistent and systematized attempt to provide ongoing bibliographic coverage of medical materials from all countries.

2.11 *Index-Catalogue of the Library of the Surgeon-General's Office.* Ser. 1–5. Washington, DC, Government Printing Office, 1880–1961. 61 vols.

2.12 *Index Medicus: A Monthly Classified Record of the Current Medical Literature of the World.* Ser. 1–3. Various publishers, 1879–1927. 45 vols.

Both book and periodical literature were included in the *Index-Catalogue*, which first began publication in 1880: all the monographic and periodical literature received by what was then the Library of the Surgeon-General's Office and which became successively the Army Medical Library, the Armed Forces Medical Library, and the National Library of Medicine.

The *Index-Catalogue* appeared in five series from 1880 to 1961. Each series contained a single alphabet, with author and subject entries appearing in dictionary form. Entries for monographs were listed under both authors' names and subject headings; periodical articles were entered only under subject headings. Items were included in the *Index-Catalogue* as they were acquired by the Library; thus, many older items may be found in later series of the work. Including all the series, more than 500,000 monographs and 2,500,000 journal articles are listed. (Journal articles were dropped in later series.)

It must be remembered that the set is the catalog of one library and as such is a record of the holdings of that library. The catalog thus is not a complete medical bibliography; however, the comprehensiveness of the collection that eventually became the National Library of Medicine causes this catalog to be the most extensive record available of the medical literature of the period.

The importance of the *Index-Catalogue* was great in its time, and it is still considered a valuable retrospective bibliography to have in any large medical or university library. Because of the early works that have been included, it is a valuable historical source.

Since each successive series was being published over a period of many years, it was necessary to have some means of bringing the *Index-Catalogue* up to date. For this purpose, Billings created the *Index Medicus,* which was published from 1879 to 1927 (with several breaks). It contained entries for both books and journal articles and included many entries not found elsewhere. Its arrangement was by subject with an author index, and it was published first monthly, then quarterly.

2.13 National Library of Medicine. *Catalog, 1948–1965.* Washington, DC, Library of Congress. Annual; five-year cumulations, beginning 1950/54–65.

From 1948 until 1965, these volumes were published as a supplement to the printed catalogs being issued by LC. They also serve as a bridge for monographs between the final series of the *Index-Catalogue,* which covered monographs published up to 1950, and the *National Library of Medicine Current Catalog,* the printed catalog derived from the CATLINE data base. Each volume includes cataloging information for monographs cataloged during the period, regardless of the date of publication.

2.14 *National Union Catalog: Pre-1956 Imprints.* London, Mansell. 1968– . Scheduled for completion in 1980; approximately 660 vols.

The Library of Congress's cumulative publication of its printed catalogs prior to 1956, plus previously unpublished material located in the *National Union Catalog,* represents another significant source of information about older monographic publications and serial titles in the health sciences. *Pre-56 Imprints* contains, in one alphabet, entries for materials published prior to January 1, 1956, that have been cataloged by the LC or by one of the participating libraries in the *NUC*. When completed, it will comprise one of the largest sets of printed materials in the world.

REFERENCES

[1]Katz, William A. *Introduction to Reference Work*. 3d ed. New York, NY, McGraw-Hill, 1978. Vol. I, p. 33.
[2]Brodman, Estelle. *The Development of Medical Bibliography*. Baltimore, MD, Medical Library Association, 1954.

READINGS

Brodman, Estelle. *The Development of Medical Bibliography*. Baltimore, MD, Medical Library Association, 1954.
Grogan, Denis. Bibliographies. In: *Science and Technology: An Introduction to the Literature*. 3d ed., rev. London, Clive Bingley, 1976.
Katz, William A. Bibliographies: National Library Catalogs and Trade Bibliographies. In: *Introduction to Reference Work, Volume One: Basic Information Sources*. 3d ed. New York, NY, McGraw-Hill, 1978. pp. 55–94.
Sutherland, F. M. Indexes, Abstracts, Bibliographies and Reviews. In: Morton, L. T. *Use of Medical Literature*. 2d ed. London, Butterworths, 1977. pp. 39–61.

CHAPTER 3

Bibliographic Sources
for
Periodicals

FRED W. ROPER

In most health sciences libraries, the periodicals collection constitutes the major element of the library's holdings. Thus, there is a strong need for tools that assist in the identification and verification of periodical titles. Because no one library can ever acquire enough materials to be self-sufficient, bibliographic sources that give locations for periodicals are essential. Finally, the health sciences librarian is continuously concerned with collection development and the selection of titles to be added to or dropped from the library's holdings.

To achieve these various purposes, the librarian needs to have available in the reference collection a variety of bibliographic sources that deal primarily or in part with periodicals. Included among these sources are bibliographies of periodicals, single library holdings lists, and union catalogs—both those that specialize in the health sciences and those of a more general nature.

HISTORICAL NOTE

It was not until 1665 that the scientific periodical as a publishing form came into existence. The *Journal des Sçavans,* first published on January 5, 1665, is considered the first learned journal. Soon after the initial appearance of the *Journal,* the Royal Society (London) began publication of the *Philosophical Transactions of the Royal Society.* The *Journal* was aimed at the amateur, while the *Philosophical Transactions* was intended to serve as a "means of communication between practising scientists, as well as a journal of interesting and curious knowledge."[1]

From these beginnings in the seventeenth century, the number of scientific periodicals has increased at an extremely rapid rate, particularly since the mid-twentieth century. The periodical has now become the vehicle for first publication of research results and for quicker communication with colleagues. To the book, on the other hand, has been relegated the task of "the formal and proper publication of mature reflections or a completed *opus* . . ." rather than the reporting of work currently in progress.[2]

CURRENT SOURCES

Because of the many vagaries associated with periodicals, bibliographic work with them can be a challenge to the librarian. Changes are constantly taking place: title variations, publishing pattern and format changes, cessations, and "rebirths" are only a few of the possibilities.

The sheer number of periodical publications makes it difficult for the librarian to be aware of what is being and has been published. The large number of titles stems partly from the "publish-or-perish" syndrome and partly from spin-offs of periodicals, creating new and separate titles. A related problem occurs when authors submit either the same article or reworked material to more than one publication.

A variety of sources is available to help the librarian to remain informed about the status of currently published periodicals. Of primary importance to health sciences librarians is the National Library of Medicine's (NLM) SERLINE and CATLINE systems and their by-products.

3.1 SERLINE (*SER*ials on *LINE*). Bethesda, MD, National Library of Medicine.

3.2 *Index of NLM Serial Titles.* 2d ed. Bethesda, MD, National Library of Medicine, 1979.

3.3 *Health Sciences Serials.* Bethesda, MD, National Library of Medicine. 1978– . Quarterly.

3.4 CATLINE (*CAT* alog on *LINE*). Bethesda, MD, National Library of Medicine.

3.5 *National Library of Medicine Current Catalog.* Bethesda, MD, National Library of Medicine. 1966– . Quarterly; annual and five-year cumulations.

The first-named source, SERLINE, is a record of all serials and congresses on order or currently received by NLM plus a small number of titles not held by NLM. There are approximately 33,000 titles in the data base, and titles in the NLM collection that are no longer being published are being added. Through the addition of location symbols for approximately 120 resource libraries in the Regional Medical Library Network, SERLINE serves as both a bibliographic record and a source of location information for interlibrary loan work.

A new SERLINE product, *Health Sciences Serials*, began in 1979. This quarterly publication, which is distributed in microfiche, contains the same information as the SERLINE data base, including location information for approximately 120 other medical libraries in the Regional Medical Library Network.

The *Index of NLM Serial Titles* is also produced from the SERLINE data base. The current edition contains 31,000 entries, representing both current and ceased serials in the NLM collection: "The *Index* is designed to assist librarians in the rapid identification of biomedical serials and to provide the necessary information for requesting serial interlibrary loans from the National Library of Medicine." Very brief information is provided: title, International Standard Serial Number (ISSN), and NLM call number. For further bibliographic information, other sources need to be consulted.

A new NLM publication in 1980 will be *List of Serials and Monographs Indexed for Online Users*. One section will consist of a single alphabetical list of all title abbreviations of all the serials in the MEDLINE file; the Health, Planning, and Administration File; and the upcoming POPLINE file. It will include the same elements of information as presently found in the abbreviations section of *List of Journals Indexed in Index Medicus* (LJI) including the NLM call number. If the title is not an *Index Medicus* title, there will be an indication as to which file it belongs. A second section will be a title listing of all monographs indexed in the current year plus the two previous ones. The new publication will serve as a bridge between the online data bases and the available printed tools.

In chapter 2, CATLINE was described as a source of information about monographs and serials that have been cataloged or recataloged at NLM since 1965. The 32,000 serials in the CATLINE file do not necessarily overlap with SERLINE. However, the information given in CATLINE represents full cataloging information.

The printed catalog, *National Library of Medicine Current Catalog,* derived from the CATLINE data base, contains cataloging data, arranged both by subject and by main entry, for NLM serials cataloged since 1965.

3.6 *Medical Books and Serials in Print.* New York, NY, Bowker. 1978– . Annual.

Included in *Medical Books and Serials in Print* is an international listing of "selected titles of periodicals issued more frequently than once a year and usually published at regular intervals, and of irregular serials and annuals provided the last issue date was not earlier than 1968" (p. vii). The entries have been taken from the same data base used to compile Bowker's *Ulrich's International Periodicals Directory, Irregular Serials and Annuals,* and *Ulrich's Quarterly.* Each of these more general titles will be of value to the medical librarian because of the wide range of periodicals beyond the health sciences likely to be included in the library's collection.

3.7   *Ulrich's International Periodicals Directory.* New York, NY, Bowker. 1932– . Biennial.

3.8   *Irregular Serials and Annuals: An International Directory.* 5th ed. New York, NY, Bowker, 1978.

3.9   *Ulrich's Quarterly.* New York, NY, Bowker. 1977– . Quarterly.

3.10   *Sources of Serials.* New York, NY, Bowker, 1977.

Ulrich's International Periodicals Directory and *Irregular Serials and Annuals* together provide information on almost 100,000 titles currently being published throughout the world. *Ulrich's* covers titles published more frequently than once a year, and *Irregular Serials and Annuals* includes titles issued annually or less frequently than once a year, or irregularly. Both publications are biennial, and *Ulrich's Quarterly* serves as the means to update them between editions. The *Quarterly,* which began publication in 1977, includes new titles with sections for changes that have occurred: a title-change index and a listing of cessations.

Source of Serials serves as a companion to the above-mentioned titles and provides an international name authority file for all serial publishers and corporate authors included in them. Included are "63,000 publishers and corporate authors arranged under 181 countries, listing 90,000 current serial titles they publish or sponsor" (Preface).

Lists from Indexing and Abstracting Services

The major indexing and abstracting services in the health sciences provide lists of the periodicals they index and abstract on a regular basis, and these lists serve as important supplements to the more inclusive bibliographies of current periodicals.

3.11 *List of Journals Indexed in Index Medicus.* Bethesda, MD, National Library of Medicine. 1960– .

3.12 Excerpta Medica. *List of Journals Abstracted.* Amsterdam, Excerpta Medica Foundation. 1964– . Annual.

3.13 *BIOSIS List of Serials.* Philadelphia, PA, Biosciences Information Service. Annual.

3.14 Science Citation Index. *Guide and Lists of Source Publications.* Philadelphia, PA, Institute for Scientific Information. Annual.

3.15 *Chemical Abstracts Service Source Index.* Columbus, OH, Chemical Abstracts Service, 1969. *Quarterly Supplement.* 1970– . Quarterly; cumulated annually.

Journals that have been selected by the National Library of Medicine for indexing in *Index Medicus* are those that have been judged to be the most useful to *Index Medicus* users; at present more than 2,500 journals are included. The *List of Journals Indexed in Index Medicus* arranges these titles in four sections: abbreviated title, full title, subject field, and country of origin. In addition, information is provided on additions, deletions, and changes. The *List* is kept up to date in the monthly *Index Medicus.* Beginning with the 1980 *List,* the NLM call number will be included.

The Excerpta Medica *List of Journals Abstracted* is also an annual publication, which in the future will be prepared from the EM data base. Between editions, there is another full list available on microfiche. The microfiche list provides, in addition to bibliographic information, the frequency of article selection from each journal included over the past twelve months.[3]

The *BIOSIS List of Serials* contains entries for more than 12,000 titles—those presently being covered in the BIOSIS products and archival entries no longer being actively covered. The preface states that the latter "have been retained to enhance the value of the list as a reference work." Additional sections include information on changes that have taken place for individual titles.

The *Science Citation Index* publication provides a guide to the use of the index and a section listing the serial publications covered in *SCI,* arranged by abbreviation, publisher, full title, subject, and country of origin. It also includes a list of the multiauthored books indexed for *SCI.*

The *Chemical Abstracts Service Source Index (CASSI)* includes information on titles included in the various CAS services and provides a variety of other types of information. Appearing on a quarterly basis, *CASSI* provides complete bibliographic information plus location information for the CAS titles in major libraries. In this way *CASSI* functions both as a complete source of bibliographic information and as a union catalog.

Library and Union Lists

Sources that reveal library holdings of periodicals are essential in locating the nearest centers for borrowing or for photocopying desired articles. These bibliographies fall into two categories: lists for single libraries and those that give the holdings for a number of libraries.

Good examples of health sciences periodicals holdings lists for single libraries are those prepared by NLM and the University of California at Los Angeles (UCLA) Biomedical Library.

3.16 *Index of NLM Serial Titles.* 2d ed. Bethesda, MD, National Library of Medicine, 1979.

3.17 UCLA Biomedical Library. *Serials Holdings List.* 6th rev. ed. Los Angeles, CA, University of California, 1977.

Although the NLM *Index* has previously been discussed, it is appropriate to note again the importance of this list for interlibrary loan work. Because of the size of the periodicals collection at NLM, the *Index* provides a tremendous resource in attempting to locate materials. More than 30,000 titles are represented in this by-product of SERLINE.

The UCLA list represents another large collection in the health sciences and offers access to periodicals in the biological sciences as well. More than 13,000 titles are included in the 1977 list, and of these, more than half are current titles to which the library has subscriptions. Included in the information for each title are complete holdings records.

Other libraries also publish individual lists, with variations as to the intent of each list and the amount of information offered. These lists will range from current subscription lists to catalogs of all titles held by the library, ceased and current, with complete holdings information. As aids to bibliographic verification and location, they are indispensable in a reference collection, and the reference librarian needs to be aware of local and regional lists that can be of immediate assistance.

Union lists range from national lists to regional and local union catalogs that reveal holdings within an area. Examples of city and state union lists follow.

3.18 Medical Library Center of New York. *Union Catalog of Medical Periodicals.* New York, NY, Medical Library Center. 1966– . Quarterly since 1976.

3.19 *North Carolina Union List of Biomedical Serials.* 4th ed. Durham, NC, Duke University Medical Center Library, 1978.

The *Union Catalog of Medical Periodicals* represents the holdings of 200 libraries in Region II (New York and New Jersey). Included are approximately 54,000 periodical titles; in addition to holdings information, there are bibliographic notes giving the history of each title with dates and frequency of publication.

The *North Carolina Union List of Biomedical Serials* contains the listings of eight biomedical libraries in North Carolina and provides information in a format similar to the *Union Catalog of Medical Periodicals.* These lists for two disparate areas—one the largest metropolitan area in the country and the other a state where the medical libraries are widely scattered—are but two of the lists of this type. It is the practice with smaller hospital libraries in a close geographic area to create a union list to facilitate resource sharing and maximize the use of the collections.

In addition to those lists that are oriented to the health sciences, a number of more general union lists should be noted.

3.20 *New Serial Titles.* Washington, DC, Library of Congress. 1953– . Eight issues per year; cumulated quarterly and annually.

3.21 *New Serial Titles: A Union List of Serials Commencing Publication After December 31, 1949; 1950–1970 Cumulative.* New York, NY, Bowker, 1973. 4 vols. *New Serial Titles, 1950–1970 Subject Guide.* New York, NY, Bowker, 1975. 2 vols.

3.22 *Union List of Serials in Libraries of the United States and Canada.* 3d ed. New York, NY, H. W. Wilson, 1965. 5 vols.

3.23 *World List of Scientific Periodicals Published in the Years 1900– 1960.* 4th ed. Washington, DC, Butterworths, 1963.

3.24 *British Union-Catalogue of Periodicals.* New York, NY, Academic Press, 1955. *Supplement to 1960.* New York, NY, Academic Press, 1962.

3.25 *British Union-Catalogue of Periodicals: New Periodical Titles.* London, Butterworths. 1964– . Quarterly; cumulated annually.

New Serial Titles, produced by the Library of Congress (LC), reflects the titles reported by LC or by one of the participating libraries in the National Union Catalog. It is intended to provide bibliographic and holdings information of serials that have begun publication since 1950, and as such it serves as a supplement to the *Union List of Serials.* It appears in eight monthly issues with four quarterly issues cumulating the two previous months and including the current one. These issues in turn appear as an annual cumulation, with longer cumulations over five- and ten-year periods. (A twenty-year cumulation, 1950–70, was published in 1973.) As libraries continue to report a title, new locations are listed in each succeeding cumulation. For titles that began publication prior to 1950, the *Union List of Serials* must be consulted.

These two titles give extensive coverage to periodicals from all countries, in all languages, and in all subject areas so long as the periodicals are held by a library in the United States or Canada that reports its holdings.

In Great Britain, two titles of importance are the *World List of Scientific Periodicals* and the *British Union-Catalogue of Periodicals.* The fourth edition of the *World List,* which appeared from 1963 to 1965, covers scientific, technical, and medical periodicals published from 1900 to 1960 that are held in British libraries. The *British Union-Catalogue of Periodicals* and its supplement cover periodicals from the seventeenth century to 1960 from all over the world in all subject areas so long as they are held in reporting British libraries. These two publications are now kept current through the computer-produced quarterly publication, *New Periodical Titles,* published by the *British Union Catalogue of Periodicals* and uniting that publication with the *World List of Scientific Periodicals.* It appears quarterly and cumulates annually into two volumes. One volume covers *all* titles included in the quarterly issues, and the other includes *only* the scientific, technical, and medical entries. This latter publication serves as the on-going continuation of the *World List of Scientific Periodicals.*

The *Chemical Abstracts Service Source Index* represents another important union list in the sciences. Not only does *Chemical Abstracts Service Source Index 1907–1974 Cumulative* include locations of periodicals indexed by the Chemical Abstracts Service (CAS), but it also covers those indexed by Engineering Index, the Institute for Scientific Information, and the BioSciences Information Service of Biological Abstracts (BIOSIS). The *CASSI Quarterly Supplement* carries location information only for those publications indexed by CAS.

ABBREVIATIONS

The reference librarian is often asked to aid in the identification of abbreviations of periodical titles, usually from a bibliography in a monograph or periodical article. The major problem associated with this aspect of work with periodicals is the lack of standardization observed in the formulation of the abbreviations. Although standards have been developed by the American National Standards Institute (Z39 Subcommittee on Periodical Title Abbreviations), actual practice continues to vary.

Lack of regard for standardization has led to similar abbreviations for different titles and to different abbreviations for the same title. Each of the lists of titles indexed by the major indexing services includes an approach by abbreviation. In addition to these titles, *World List of Scientific Periodicals* and the *British Union Catalogue of Periodicals* also offer access by abbreviation.

When the same abbreviation is used for two or more titles, further detective work will be necessary to determine which title is meant. The publishing history of the titles will have to be examined, and a source that provides complete bibliographic information will need to be consulted; SERLINE, the *Union Catalog of Medical Periodicals, Ulrich's International Periodicals Directory, Union List of Serials, New Serial Titles, World List of Scientific Periodicals, British Union-Catalogue of Periodicals,* and *Chemical Abstracts Service Source Index* will be of particular value.

CHANGES

One of the challenges of periodicals work is keeping up with the changes that take place in the bibliographic record of a periodical. The most common changes are births (new publications), deaths (cessations), and title changes. Obviously any element in the bibliographic record may change, but these are the major problem areas.

   3.26 *Vital Notes on Medical Periodicals.* New York, NY, Medical Library Association. 1952– . Three times per year.

Vital Notes on Medical Periodicals, a publication of the Medical Library Association, deals specifically with these kinds of problems. It is produced at the Medical Library Center of New York "as a closely related task to the maintenance of two computer-based serials projects processed in house: The PHILSOM automated serials control system, and the *Union Catalog of Medical Periodicals* data base" (Preface).

Vital Notes depends heavily on participating libraries for the material that is included. Currency is stressed, and bibliographic activity and changes are recorded for the current year plus the two preceding years.

Additional sources that have special sections to note changes in periodical information include *Ulrich's International Periodicals Directory, Ulrich's Quarterly, List of Journals Indexed in Index Medicus, BIOSIS List of Serials, Chemical Abstracts Service Source Index, New Serial Titles,* and *New Periodical Titles.*

REFERENCES

[1]Brodman, Estelle. *The Development of Medical Bibliography.* Baltimore, MD, Medical Library Association, 1954. pp. 49–50.
[2]Grogan, Denis. *Science and Technology: An Introduction to the Literature.* 3d ed., rev. London, Clive Bingley, 1976. p. 126.
[3]Excerpta Medica. *List of Journals Abstracted.* Amsterdam, Excerpta Medica Foundation, 1979. Preface.

READINGS

Grogan, Denis. Perodicals. In: *Science and Technology: An Introduction to the Literature.* 3d ed., rev. London, Clive Bingley, 1976. pp. 126–168.
Houghton, Bernard. *Scientific Periodicals: Their Historical Development, Characteristics and Control.* London, Clive Bingley, 1975.
Katz, William A. *Introduction to Reference Work, Volume One: Basic Information Sources.* 3d ed. New York, NY, McGraw-Hill, 1978. pp. 77–81.
Kronick, David A. *A History of Scientific and Technical Periodicals: The Origins and Development of the Scientific and Technical Press, 1665–1790.* 2d ed. Metuchen, NJ, Scarecrow, 1976.

CHAPTER 4

Indexing
and
Abstracting Services

JO ANNE BOORKMAN

Indexing and abstracting services are designed to provide access to periodical and other literature through a variety of approaches. Subjects, in the form of either keywords or thesaurus terms, are frequently used as access points; however, approaches by authors and cited authors* are also possible. An index provides the basic bibliographic information needed to locate an article: author(s) name, article title, journal title, journal volume and year, and pages of the article. An abstracting service provides the same information but in addition includes a brief summary of an article's content—an abstract.

Indexing and abstracting services vary widely in the way they provide access to the bibliographic information they are presenting. It is, therefore, important to evaluate the services by criteria that will give an idea of their value to us and their ease of use.

In using these services to help requesters develop bibliographies, verify references, and find information, it is essential to know the scope and coverage of each service. Not only is subject coverage important to note, but also the depth of coverage and the types of materials indexed—journals, books, dissertations, government documents, etc. If a journal is indexed, are all the articles included? Or just selected ones? Are brief reports indexed? Substantive letters to the editor? The number of serials indexed should also be noted, as well as languages and time period covered.

The number and types of indexes can vary with the scope and type of material covered by a service. Subject and author indexes are generally found in all, while report number, patent, molecular for-

---

*An author listed in the bibliography of an article or book.

mula, systematic and citation indexes are found in specialized abstracting and indexing services. Some author indexes list only the first author of a paper, while others include additional authors. It is important to know the policy of an index as to whether all an author's writings will be listed or just the ones for which he or she is the primary author.

Subject indexes take all sorts of forms. Some subject indexes are strictly keyword indexes created by extracting terms from the title of an article, while others augment the keywords from titles with additional terms provided by indexers. In still other instances the indexes use a controlled vocabulary or thesaurus where subject descriptors are assigned by indexers to describe the content of the article referenced. Whether a strictly defined term must be used to look up articles on a subject (e.g., the *Medical Subject Headings* with *Index Medicus*) or a variety of synonyms are provided to cover that subject (the *Permuterm Subject Index* of *Science Citation Index*) will make a big difference in the analysis of a bibliographic question. The choice of initial index is often based on how easily the subject can be searched when one uses the structure of the subject index.

Two types of keyword indexes that should be mentioned are the KWIC and KWOC indexes. A KWIC (Keyword in Content) index takes keywords as they appear in the title of an article and lists the title in the index alphabetically under each significant word. An augmented KWIC index would include terms selected from the abstract by an indexer. An example of this type of index is that used by the Bio-Sciences Information Service of Biological Abstracts (BIOSIS) in the subject index to *Biological Abstracts.* The KWOC (Keyword out of Content) index employs all significant words from the title and does not list them with the title, but instead refers to the complete citation by reference number or author's name. For example, a listing from the *Permuterm Subject Index* for *Science Citation Index* would look like this:

> Root
> canal—Miyoshi S
> Nevins A

In some services the indexes are very brief in the monthly or quarterly issues, as the services prefer to list citations by broad subject classification, limiting detailed indexes to semiannual or annual cumulations.

The arrangement of the information can vary widely in both indexes and abstracts. The sequence of bibliographic elements for an entry as well as where the unit entry* is listed should be noted. Unit entries can be listed in a classified, author, subject, or journal title arrangement, to name the most commonly used formats. Generally the indexes arrange citations directly under author or subject or both, as in *Index Medicus*. Abstracting services as a rule arrange the citations with abstracts in a classified or broad subject arrangement with author, detailed subject, and special indexes referring to the citation or reference number in the classified section. *Excerpta Medica* and *Biological Abstracts* both follow this format. If foreign-language articles are indexed, the language that the title appears in should be noted. For translated titles, the language of the article should be indicated. In an index, the availability of an English abstract in the journal is also noteworthy. For further assessment of an abstracting service, the source of an abstract, signed, anonymous, or from the journal, can indicate whether the abstract is critical or simply a summary of the article. Generally, signed abstracts are written by subject specialists and are more critical than author abstracts.

Publication characteristics of the service should also be considered. What is the average time between the publication of an original article and its appearance in an indexing or abstracting journal? The frequency of publication of the indexing or abstracting service has some bearing on the time lag associated with a citation's appearance. However, abstracting services tend to have a longer time lag than indexing services.

The value of any indexing or abstracting service will also depend on how easy it is to use. However, even complicated formats can be helpful, provided the service gives information on how best to use its product. Therefore, a further criterion to look for is whether the service has provided a guide to using the index or abstracting source, a list of journals, other material covered by the service, and a list of journal title abbreviations.

Another factor to consider is the cost of the service, not just in relation to the library budget but also in relation to the other indexing and abstracting services in a library's collection. In this context, uniqueness of coverage should be weighed against overlap of coverage. The service's usefulness as a reference tool in terms of the needs of the library's primary clientele must be considered as well.

Unit entry is defined as the entry where the complete bibliographic reference is listed.

In the following review of the major indexing and abstracting services in the health sciences, the above criteria will be used: coverage, access to information, arrangement of information, and publication characteristics. Some libraries will undoubtedly also have to weigh the usefulness of these tools to their clientele against budgetary constraints. The printed versions of these services are discussed in this chapter. The online data bases and their capabilities will be discussed in the following chapter.

INDEX MEDICUS

4.1 *Index Medicus*. Bethesda, MD, National Library of Medicine. Vol. 1– , 1960– .

The *Index Medicus* is the major index to medical periodical literature. The *Index Medicus* (New Series) began in 1960. Its predecessors— beginning with the *Index-Catalogue of the Library of the Surgeon General's Office*, United States Army, vol. 1, 1880, and *Index Medicus*, vol. 1, 1879, and followed by the *Quarterly Cumulative Index to Current Medical Literature*—will not be discussed here (see figure 4–1). A brief history of these publications and their relationship to one another is in the Introduction to *Cumulated Index Medicus*, vol. 1, 1960.[1,2]

Index Medicus (IM) appears monthly and cumulates annually. The first five cumulative volumes (vols. 1–5, 1960–64) were published by the American Medical Association (AMA) with subsequent cumulative volumes published by the National Library of Medicine (NLM). The current index is broad in coverage, indexing more than 2,500 journals in the medical and health-related sciences as well as selected monographs and conference proceedings (since May 1976) from the international literature. Approximately half the citations refer to articles in languages other than English, indicated by brackets around the English translation of the title with the original language noted at the end of the citation. In the early 1960s NLM began developing its computerized bibliographic data base, the *MEDical Literature Analysis and Retrieval System* (MEDLARS), for producing *Index Medicus*.[3] Since 1966 the format of *Index Medicus* has remained essentially the same.

The bulk of the index has a subject arrangement with full citations listed directly under each subject heading. Subject headings are assigned by indexers at NLM using a controlled vocabulary, *Medical Subject Headings (MeSH)*. Subject headings are further delineated by

Figure 4–1. Medical indexes to periodical literature

Index Medicus J. S. Billings, et al.	1879–99; series I 1903–20; series II 1921–27; series III	Monthly publication Indexing periodical literature

Bibliographia Medica
  Paris, Institut de
  Bibliographie
	1900–03, vols. 1–3	Covers the years between series I
		and series II of *Index Medicus*

Index Catalogue
  J. S. Billings, et al.
	1880–95; 1st series,
	        16 vols.
	1896–16; 2nd series,
	        21 vols.
	1918–32; 3rd series,
	        10 vols.
	1936–48; 4th series,
	        11 vols. (A–MEZ)
	1955; 4th series,
	        1 vol. (Mh–Mn)
	1959, 61; 5th series,
	        3 vols.
		
		Indexing monographs and periodicals
		
		Indexing monographs and periodicals
		
		Indexing monographs and periodicals
		
		Indexing monographs and periodicals
		
		Monographs only
		1959 Authors and titles only
		1961 Subjects A–M; N–Z

Quarterly Cumulative Index (QCI), AMA	1916–26; 12 volumes	Clinical journals indexed with some books and government documents
Quarterly Cumulative Index Medicus (QCIM), AMA	1927–56	Supersedes *Index Medicus* and *QCI* Army Medical Library furnished some citations until 1932
Current List of Medical Literature (CLML)	1941–59	Published privately by A. Seidell, later assisted by the Army Medical Library; in 1945 the Army Medical Library took over the publication
Index Medicus (New Series)	1960–	Took the place of the *QCIM* and superseded *CLML*

the use of subheadings. For example, an article on the anatomy of the eye would be listed in the index under EYE/anatomy and histology, and an article on the use of penicillin to treat a disease would be found under PENICILLIN/therapeutic use. Indexers are instructed to assign the most specific subject headings or subject heading/ subheading combinations to describe the *content* of an article. Therefore, it is important to determine the appropriate subject headings, by using *MeSH*, for a topic before approaching *Index Medicus*. As a further example, an article on the physiology of the retina of the eye will be indexed under RETINA/physiology but *not* EYE/physiology, since the article is on the retina, a specific part of the eye, and not the eye in general.

MeSH is revised annually, with new terms added and old terms changed to current terminology or deleted. There are four published forms of *MeSH*, to help select appropriate subject headings: an alphabetic list that appears annually as part two of the January issue of *Index Medicus*; an annotated alphabetic list (figure 4–2); a tree structure (figure 4–3), which is an hierarchical arrangement of the subject terms; and a permuted list (figure 4–4). The alphabetic *MeSH* and annotated alphabetic *MeSH* provide cross-references from terms that are *not* subject headings to *MeSH* terms, as well as to related *MeSH* terms that could be appropriate to a topic. The date the term entered the vocabulary, and tree numbers indicating in which categories the term belongs are also provided in both versions of the alphabetic *MeSH*. Notes on the usage of a term and allowable subheadings are included in the annotated *MeSH* for use by indexers, catalogers, and searchers. The *MeSH* tree structure provides a subject categorization of the vocabulary in fifteen sections, e.g., A. Anatomy, C. Diseases, D. Drugs and Chemicals, etc. Each section is further broken down for specificity. The tree structure is an important tool in helping to select terms that are not easily scanned in the alphabetic *MeSH* (see figure 4–3). It is an even more important tool for online computer searching of the MEDLARS data base, MEDLINE. In addition to its uses for indexing and manual searching of *Index Medicus* and computer searching of MEDLINE, the *MeSH* vocabulary is used for cataloging and manual searching of NLM's *Current Catalog* and *Audiovisuals Catalog* as well as computer searching of their online counterparts, CATLINE and AVLINE. It is further used by most health sciences libraries for subject cataloging of their collections for the public catalog.

Figure 4–2. Annotated Alphabetic and Alphabetic *MeSH*

Annotated Alphabetic *MeSH*	**Alphabetic *MeSH*** **(no annotations in this version)**
QUALITY ASSURANCE PROGRAM see QUALITY OF HEALTH CARE N4.761+	QUALITY ASSURANCE PROGRAM see QUALITY OF HEALTH CARE

QUALITY CONTROL
 J1.897.608
 NIM; no qualif
 74(71)
 see related
    REFERENCE STANDARDS
	QUALITY CONTROL
	 J1.897.608
	 74
	 see related
	    REFERENCE STANDARDS

QUALITY OF HEALTH CARE
 N4.761+
 only /econ /legis /trends   CATALOG: /geog /form
 68
 see related
    PROFESSIONAL STAFF COMMITTEES
    SOCIAL CONTROL, FORMAL
 X   QUALITY ASSURANCE PROGRAM
	QUALITY OF HEALTH CARE
	 N4.761+
	 68
	 see related
	    PROFESSIONAL STAFF COMMITTEES
	    SOCIAL CONTROL, FORMAL
	 X QUALITY ASSURANCE PROGRAM

QUALITY OF LIFE I1.800 K1.752.770 no qualif; consider also LIFE STYLE 77(75)	QUALITY OF LIFE I1.800 K1.752.770 77

Under QUALITY OF HEALTH CARE note:

N4.761+—*MeSH* tree number; + indicates more specific terms are listed under this number

see related—other *MeSH* terms to consider

X—Quality Assurance Programs are indexed with the term QUALITY OF HEALTH CARE

only /econ /legis /trends—indicate subheadings that can be used with this term in *Index Medicus,* listed in Annotated *MeSH* only

68—the date the term started being used in the *MeSH* vocabulary

Under QUALITY OF LIFE note:

no qualif—no subheadings are used with this term

77 (75)—77 is the date the term entered the vocabulary for use in *Index Medicus;* (75) the date indexers began using the term for online retrieval, listed in the Annotated *MeSH* only

National Library of Medicine, *Medical Subject Headings, Annotated Alphabetic List,* 1979 (Springfield, VA, National Technical Information Service, 1978), p. 541; *Medical Subject Headings, 1979 Index Medicus* 20 (1 pt 2):321, 1979.

Figure 4–3. *MeSH* Tree Structure

PRIMARY HEALTH CARE	N4.590.233.727
CONTINUITY OF PATIENT CARE⁺	N4.590.233.727.210
PROGRESSIVE PATIENT CARE	N4.590.233.799
DELIVERY OF HEALTH CARE	N4.590.374
HEALTH SERVICES ACCESSIBILITY	N4.590.374.200
PATIENT CARE TEAM	N4.590.715
NURSING, TEAM	N4.590.715.571
QUALITY OF HEALTH CARE	N4.761
MEDICAL AUDIT	N4.761.380
COMMISSION ON PROFESSIONAL AND HOSPITAL ACTIVITIES⁺	N4.761.380.100
NURSING AUDIT	N4.761.520
OUTCOME AND PROCESS ASSESSMENT (HEALTH CARE)	N4.761.559
PEER REVIEW	N4.761.610 N4.452.758.
PROFESSIONAL STANDARDS REVIEW ORGANIZATIONS	N4.761.673
UTILIZATION REVIEW	N4.761.879
CONCURRENT REVIEW⁺	N4.761.879.200

N4.761—common tree number for Quality of Health Care terms
*—indicates minor descriptors used in indexing but not used in
   the printed *Index Medicus*
N4.452.758—tree number where PEER REVIEW is also listed

National Library of Medicine, *Medical Subject Headings Tree Structure,
1979* (Springfield, VA; National Technical Information Service,
1978, pp. 422–23).

Citations are indexed with twelve to sixteen subject headings but
will be listed in the printed *Index Medicus* under three to five headings.
English-language articles are listed first (alphabetically arranged by
journal title abbreviation), and each entry includes the title, author,
journal, volume, page, and, for review articles, the number of references in the bibliography. Foreign-language citations follow, with the
language indicated in parentheses following the reference. The availability of an English abstract in the journal is also noted. The author
index provides the bibliographic reference after the first author's
name with cross-references from additional authors' names referring
to the first author.

Figure 4–4. Permuted *MeSH*

Each significant term in a subject heading *or* cross-reference is listed alphabetically, e.g., QUALITY OF HEALTH CARE would be listed under Quality, Health, and Care followed by *MeSH* heading(s) that are appropriate.

CARDIOVERSION
CARDIOVERSION see ELECTRIC COUNTERSHOCK

CARE
ACCEPTABILITY OF HEALTH CARE see PATIENT ACCEPTANCE OF HEALTH
    CARE
AFTER CARE
AMBULATORY CARE
CANCER CARE FACILITIES see under HOSPITALS, SPECIAL
CARDIAC CARE FACILITIES see under HOSPITALS, SPECIAL
CHILD CARE
CHILD DAY CARE CENTERS
COMMUNITY HEALTH CARE see COMMUNITY HEALTH SERVICES
COMPREHENSIVE DENTAL CARE
COMPREHENSIVE HEALTH CARE
CONTINUITY OF PATIENT CARE see under PRIMARY HEALTH CARE
CORONARY CARE UNITS
CRITICAL CARE
CUSTODIAL CARE
DAY CARE
DELIVERY OF HEALTH CARE
DENTAL CARE
DENTAL CARE PLANS see INSURANCE, DENTAL
DENTAL DEVICES, HOME CARE
DOMICILIARY CARE see HOME CARE SERVICES
EMERGENCY CARE see EMERGENCY HEALTH SERVICES
EXTENDED CARE FACILITIES see SKILLED NURSING FACILITIES
FOSTER HOME CARE
HEALTH CARE DELIVERY see DELIVERY OF HEALTH CARE
HEALTH CARE TEAM see PATIENT CARE TEAM
HOME CARE SERVICES
INDIGENT CARE see MEDICAL INDIGENCY
INFANT CARE
INTENSIVE CARE UNITS
INTERMEDIATE CARE FACILITIES see under NURSING HOMES
LIFE SUPPORT CARE
LONG TERM CARE
MEDICAL CARE TEAM see PATIENT CARE TEAM
MINIMAL CARE UNITS see SELF-CARE UNITS
NIGHT CARE
NURSING CARE
OUTCOME AND PROCESS ASSESSMENT (HEALTH CARE)
PASTORAL CARE
PATIENT ACCEPTANCE OF HEALTH CARE
PATIENT CARE PLANNING
PATIENT CARE TEAM
POSTNATAL CARE
POSTOPERATIVE CARE
PRENATAL CARE
PREOPERATIVE CARE
PREPAID DENTAL CARE see INSURANCE, DENTAL
PRIMARY CARE PHYSICIANS see PHYSICIANS, FAMILY
PRIMARY HEALTH CARE
PRIMARY NURSING CARE
PROGRESSIVE PATIENT CARE
QUALITY OF HEALTH CARE
RESPIRATORY CARE UNITS
ROOMING-IN CARE see under INFANT CARE
SELF CARE see ACTIVITIES OF DAILY LIVING
SELF-CARE UNITS see under HOSPITAL UNITS
TERMINAL CARE

CAREER
CAREER CHOICE see under DECISION MAKING
CAREER MOBILITY

CARFECILLIN
CARFECILLIN see under CARBENICILLIN

HEALTH
ABUSE OF HEALTH SERVICES see HEALTH SERVICES MISUSE
ACCEPTABILITY OF HEALTH CARE see PATIENT ACCEPTANCE OF HEALTH
    CARE
ACCESSIBILITY OF HEALTH SERVICES see HEALTH SERVICES
    ACCESSIBILITY

OUTCOME AND PROCESS ASSESSMENT (HEALTH CARE)
OVERUTILIZATION OF HEALTH SERVICES see HEALTH SERVICES MISUSE
PAN AMERICAN HEALTH ORGANIZATION
PATIENT ACCEPTANCE OF HEALTH CARE
PERSONAL HEALTH SERVICES
PLANNING, HEALTH AND WELFARE see HEALTH PLANNING
PLANNING, HEALTH FACILITY see HEALTH FACILITY PLANNING
PREVENTIVE HEALTH SERVICES
PRIMARY HEALTH CARE
PUBLIC HEALTH
PUBLIC HEALTH ADMINISTRATION
PUBLIC HEALTH DENTISTRY
PUBLIC HEALTH NURSING
PUBLIC HEALTH SERVICE see UNITED STATES PUBLIC HEALTH SERVICE
QUALITY OF HEALTH CARE
REGIONAL HEALTH PLANNING
REIMBURSEMENT, HEALTH INSURANCE see INSURANCE, HEALTH,
    REIMBURSEMENT
RURAL HEALTH
SCHOOL HEALTH SERVICES
SCHOOLS, HEALTH OCCUPATIONS
SCHOOLS, PUBLIC HEALTH
STATE HEALTH PLANNING AGENCIES, UNITED STATES see HEALTH
    SYSTEMS AGENCIES

QUADRUPLETS
QUADRUPLETS

QUAIL
JAPANESE QUAIL see COTURNIX
QUAIL

QUAKING
M I C E , Q U A K I N
MICE, QUAKING

QUALITY
QUALITY ASSURANCE PROGRAM see QUALITY OF HEALTH CARE
QUALITY CONTROL
QUALITY OF HEALTH CARE
QUALITY OF LIFE
VOICE QUALITY see under VOICE

QUANTUM
QUANTUM THEORY

QUARANTINE
QUARANTINE

QUARTZ
QUARTZ see under SILICA

National Library of Medicine, *Permuted Medical Subject Headings, 1979* (Springfield, VA; National Technical Information Service, 1978). pp. 51, 139–40, 254.

A special feature in *IM* is the monthly *Bibliography of Medical Reviews (BMR)* found at the beginning of each monthly *IM* and cumulated in the annual. It has the same format as the main index but provides separate access (subject and author) to lengthy and review articles. The separate author index will be dropped in the 1980 and subsequent editions. The *BMR* first appeared as a separate publication. Its cumulation (vol. 6, 1961) represents review articles from the 1955–59 *Current List of Medical Literature* and from the *Cumulated Index Medicus,* vol. 1, 1960; however, editing procedures for the cumulation resulted in some references being eliminated. Subsequent volumes (7–12, 1962–67) contain review articles from the previous years' *Cumulated Index Medicus,* vols, 2–7, 1961–66. The *BMR,* now a regular feature of both the monthly and cumulated *Index Medicus,* has listed the current year's review articles since the *CIM,* vol. 8, 1967, and the monthly *IM,* vol. 9, no. 1, Jan. 1968.

The MEDLARS files are also used to produce the *Abridged Index Medicus (AIM),* vol. 1– , 1970– . Designed to be used by the practicing physician, *AIM* provides citations to 125 English-language clinical journals. The format is similar to that of *Index Medicus,* with both author and subject indexes. *MeSH* subject headings are used, with the modification that articles are listed under main headings only in the monthly issues and under main heading/subheadings when appropriate in the annual *Cumulated Abridged Index Medicus. AIM* is an especially useful index for the smaller hospital library, which will not need the exhaustive research journal coverage of *Index Medicus.*

OTHER MEDICAL INDEXES AND ABSTRACTS

4.2 *Excerpta Medica.* Amsterdam, Excerpta Medica Foundation, 1947– . (Many sections)

4.3 *Medical Socioeconomic Research Sources.* Chicago, IL, Archive Library Department of the American Medical Association. Vol. 1–9, Jan. 1971–79. (Supersedes *Index to Medical Socioeconomic Literature,* vols. 1–9, 1962–70.)

Excerpta Medica is the major abstracting service for medical journals. Its scope is primarily human medicine and the basic sciences related to this field. While allied medical subjects (dentistry, nursing, psychology, veterinary medicine, etc.) appear in the sections, they are not the primary subject fields abstracted. Coverage is of over 4,500 journals, 3,500 of which are regularly scanned. These represent 95%

of the *Excerpta Medica* references, with monographs and dissertations representing 5%. The abstracts appear in one or more of the more than forty subject sections of *EM*. Each section has its own editor who selects the articles that will appear in that section and, further, decides whether the references will be abstracted for the printed *EM* publication or just be indexed and appear in the *EM* data base under that section's classification (EMCLASS) number. Sixty percent of the references appear in at least one printed *Excerpta Medica* section. The remaining 40% of the file is available only through online searching of EMBASE, the *Excerpta Medica* data base. The sections arrange the references with abstracts in a classified (subject) order within each section with author and detailed subject indexes. Two of the *Excerpta Medica* sections, *Drug Literature Index* and *Adverse Reactions Titles*, are indexes only and do not provide abstracts.

Subjects are indexed using *EM* controlled vocabulary, MALIMET.* The MALIMET vocabulary contains 180,000 preferred terms and 250,000 synonyms. It has recently been published on microfiche, providing public availability for the first time. There are three levels of indexing for the subject indexes. Primary terms, class A, represent main concepts discussed in an article; primary terms, class B, represent other concepts; and last, there are secondary terms that can be free text terms (i.e., eight cases, ten patients, etc.) or EMTAGS (i.e., bibliographic—review article, editorial, and commentary; anatomical—fetus, spleen; geographic—Western Europe, etc.).[4] In the printed index of an *EM* section these terms would give a rough idea of the content of an article.

A recent publication, *Guide to Excerpta Medica Classification and Indexing*, provides a brief description of each section, each section's classification scheme, and a general subject index indicating which sections should be searched for a given topic. Sections are listed numerically, with the principal section for a specific subject given in boldface type. This *Guide* is a logical first approach to *EM* for identifying appropriate sections in which to begin a search. MALIMET, unlike *MeSH*, is not designed to be a guide to the printed indexes. However, it should prove useful for online searching of EMBASE.

Excerpta Medica, because of its detailed indexing vocabulary, is often useful in locating articles on very narrow topics that do not have a specific enough subject approach in *Index Medicus*. Its abstracts are also helpful for providing English summaries of non-English-

---

*MAster LIst of MEdical Indexing Terms.

language articles. These are useful to identify, for a researcher, whether the article should be obtained or translated.

On the negative side *Excerpta Medica* is an extremely costly service for a library to purchase, house, and maintain. Subject sections, however, can be purchased separately, allowing smaller specialized libraries to purchase only those sections useful to their primary clientele.

Medical Socioeconomic Research Sources (Med Soc) is a quarterly publication that cumulates annually and is produced by the Division of Library and Archival Services staff of the AMA in cooperation with its Center for Health Services Research and Development and Electronic Data Processing Section. The index selectively covers English-language books, journal articles, pamphlets, unpublished speeches, theses, and selected newspaper articles in the sociology and economics of medicine. Other specific areas included are the following: education, ethics, international relations, legislation, political science, public health, religion, and statistics as they relate to medicine.

The main index lists citations under subject headings based on *MeSH* but adapted to the subject areas covered in *Med Soc*. Broad subjects are arranged in an hierarchical arrangement using subheadings. The author index lists the citation under the first author's name, with cross-references from the second and third authors only. The index is helpful in identifying articles with statistical information. It is, also, especially useful for locating material from less technical sources for less sophisticated medical library users. Unfortunately, this index ceased publication in 1979.

Nursing Indexes

4.4 *International Nursing Index*. New York, NY, American Journal of Nursing Company, in cooperation with the National Library of Medicine. Vol. 1– , 1966– .

4.5 *Cumulative Index to Nursing and Allied Health Literature*. Glendale, CA, Glendale Adventist Medical Center. Vol. 22– , 1977– . (Called *Cumulative Index to Nursing Literature*, vol. 1–21, 1956–76.)

4.6 Henderson, V. *Nursing Studies Index; an annotated guide to reported studies, research in progress, research methods, and historical materials in periodicals, books and pamphlets in English*. Vols. 1–4, 1900–59. Philadelphia, PA, Lippincott, 1963–72.

The *International Nursing Index (INI)* appears quarterly and has a format identical to that of the *Index Medicus,* with subject and author indexes. The *MeSH* vocabulary is used for the subject index. An annotated list of subject headings used in nursing as well as a list of the more than 200 journals indexed (not all are indexed by *Index Medicus*) appear as part II of the first issue of each year.

Journal coverage is international in scope and includes nursing articles from non-nursing journals gleaned from the MEDLARS system. Original signed articles, editorials of national and international interest, and biographies and obituaries of substance comprise the coverage, as well as reports of national and international organizations. Special sections in the index include a "List of Nursing Books" and a "List of Publications of Organizations and Agencies."

The *Cumulative Index to Nursing and Allied Health Literature (CINAHL)* appears in five bimonthly issues and a cumulated annual volume. It has separate author and subject indexes. (Prior to 1967 authors and subjects were in a single alphabetical listing.) Many journal article references indicate type of article in parentheses following the citation, i.e., "research," "research, nurs.," etc. Nursing students often find these notations quite helpful. Separate indexes provide references to pamphlets, audiovisuals, and book reviews.

Over 260 journals are regularly scanned, using essentially the same criteria as *INI*. In addition, the *CINAHL* indexes all serials published by the American Nurses Association, the National League for Nursing, and the DHEW Division of Nursing. Additional journals covered in an issue are listed when they appear. These often include such popular and news magazines as *Newsweek, Parents',* and *McCall's.*

The *CINAHL* regularly includes approximately 120 journals not indexed in *INI.* On the other hand, it does not have the non-nursing journal coverage that *INI* gets from MEDLARS. The two indexes thus complement each other, even though the core nursing literature is covered by both.

The *Nursing Studies Index,* compiled by the Yale University School of Nursing Index staff, provides retrospective coverage of the English-language nursing literature in a subject arrangement. Subjects are subdivided by both geographic subheadings and general subheadings, such as evaluations, manuals, etc. An author index is also provided.

Dental Indexes and Abstracts

4.7 *Index to Dental Literature.* Chicago, IL, American Dental Association and National Library of Medicine. 1962– . (Called *Index to Dental Literature in the English Language,* 1839/75–1961.)

4.8 *Dental Abstracts; a selection of world dental literature.* Chicago, IL, American Dental Association. Vol. 1– , 1956– .

4.9 *Oral Research Abstracts.* Chicago, IL, American Dental Association. Vols. 1–13, 1966–78.

The *Index to Dental Literature (IDL)* is the primary index to dental literature. It is international in scope and includes both dental journals and references to related articles from nondental journals in the MEDLARS files. Each issue of the index, which appears quarterly, includes the journals indexed for the issue. Issues cumulate into an annual volume.

Criteria for inclusion of an article are similar to that for the nursing indexes: original signed articles, editorials of national and international interest, reports of national and international organizations, and selected bibliographies. A list of dental descriptors gives cross-references and refers the user to *MeSH* for a complete subject heading listing. *MeSH* subheadings with definitions are included but are called "qualifiers." The subject index is in the same format as *Index Medicus,* as is the author index. A separate "List of New Dental Books" and a subject and author listing of "Dental Dissertations and Theses" are also included. The preface gives a concise explanation of the index, how it is constructed, and how to use it.

Dental Abstracts appears monthly and abstracts approximately 1,000 journal articles from the world literature. It provides a classified listing by broad subject and gives author and subject indexes only in the annual cumulated volume. As with many abstracting services, there is a four- to seven-month time lag between the publication of the article in a journal and its appearance in *Dental Abstracts.* Another distinct disadvantage of this publication is that it does not provide a list of the journals it abstracts.

Oral Research Abstracts also appeared monthly but was broader in scope than *Dental Abstracts* and included both dental and nondental journals. Its purpose was "to bring the facts to their [dentists'] desks and permit selective reading of original reports."[5] Approximately 7,200 signed abstracts appear annually, taken from over 1,000 journals (not listed) and patents from the world literature. There is a classified arrangement, with an author index in the monthly issues and subject and author indexes in the annual cumulated volume. Abstracts are more descriptive than critical.

Hospital Indexes and Abstracts

4.10 *Hospital Literature Index.* Chicago, IL, American Hospital Association, in cooperation with the National Library of Medicine. Vol. 11– , 1955– . (Called *Hospital Periodical Literature Index*, vols. 1–10, 1945–54.)

4.11 *Hospital Abstracts; a monthly survery of world literature.* London, Department of Health and Social Security. Jan. 1961— . (Called Ministry of Health, Jan. 1961—Nov. 1978.)

4.12 *Abstracts of Health Care Management Studies.* Ann Arbor, MI, University of Michigan, Cooperative Information Center for Health Care Management Studies. Vol. 15— , 1979— . (Called *Abstracts of Hospital Management Studies*, vols. 1—14, 1964—78.)

The *Hospital Literature Index (HLI)* has gone through several changes prior to its present format as a quarterly publication in cooperation with the National Library of Medicine; it now uses the MEDLARS system. Earlier titles—*Index to Current Hospital Literature,* vols. 1–10, 1945–54; *Hospital Periodical Literature Index,* vols. 11–13(1), 1955–June 1957; and *Hospital Literature Index,* 1957–77—were regularly compiled into six five-year cumulations as *Cumulative Index to Hospital Literature* (1945–49, 1950–54, 1955–59, 1960–64, 1965–69, 1970–74) and a final multiyear volume for 1975–77. Subsequent cumulations under MEDLARS will appear annually, similar to those of the *International Nursing Index.*

The *Hospital Literature Index* covers English-language journal literature related to the administrative aspects of the delivery of health care in hospitals, health centers, health maintenance organizations (HMOs), and other group practice facilities. Also included are articles related to nursing homes, rehabilitation centers, etc. Clinical medicine and the clinical aspects of patient care are not covered in this index, but articles on the quality of patient care can be found.

The present format of *HLI* is like that of *Index Medicus,* with citations listed directly under the subject headings as well as by the first author's name in the author index. *MeSH* (with an expanded vocabulary in hospital management and planning) is now used for subject headings in *HLI*. This supersedes Alice Dunlap's *Hospital Literature Subject Headings* (2d ed., 1977, Chicago, IL, American Hospital Association), which should be used for subject access to the cumulative indexes. The recent publication, *Hospital Literature Subject Headings Transition Guide to Medical Subject Headings* (Chicago, IL, American Hospital Association, 1978), has been designed to aid in the shift in subject heading coverage necessitated by conversion to the MEDLARS system.

In addition to the primary subject and author indexes, *HLI* provides a list of journals indexed by journal title abbreviation. A special section provides listings of books, monographs, and journals recently received by the Asa S. Bacon Library of the American Hospital Association in the following three sections: *MeSH* subject arrangement of books, reference books, and periodicals.

A monthly British publication, *Hospital Abstracts* provides abstracts to articles of all aspects of hospitals and hospital administration. Indexing is selective for nonmedical journals. Only 1,891 abstracts were provided in 1978; however, more than half the journals are not covered in *Index Medicus*. References are arranged in broad subject categories and hospital departments. Monthly issues provide only an author index, with the cumulated annual volume having both subject and author indexes. A list of addresses for publishers is also included.

Abstracts of Health Care Management Studies provides an approach to a somewhat different body of literature. Published by the Cooperative Information Center for Health Care Management Studies of the University of Michigan, it provides abstracts to management, planning, and public policies related to the delivery of health care. Both published and unpublished studies as well as those with limited distribution are abstracted.

The abstracts are arranged in a classified format of forty categories with author and subject indexes. Signed abstracts include bibliographic information and availability and ordering information for unpublished studies. A specialized index, the Source of Reference Index (SORIN), lists the sources of abstracted studies, including research agencies, sites of studies, universities, foundations, sponsoring government agencies, and journals. A list of journals gives routinely scanned sources with publishers, addresses, etc. A microfilm index lists those items available in that format from University Microfilms International.

OTHER RELATED INDEXES AND ABSTRACTS

4.13 *Biological Abstracts*. Philadelphia, PA, Union of American Biological Societies. Vol. 1– , 1926– . Biweekly.

4.14 *Bioresearch Index*. Philadelphia, PA, Biosciences Information Service of Biological Abstracts. Vol. 3– , 1967– . Monthly. (Called *Bioresearch Titles*, vols. 1 and 2, 1965–66.)

Biological Abstracts (BA) and *Bioresearch Index (BIOI)* should be used in conjunction for searching all types of literature in the life sciences. Biosciences Information Service (BIOSIS) has designed them so that the same reference is rarely cited in both. Each biweekly issue of *BA* contains abstracts to original article research papers (arranged under approximately 580 broad subject specialities), reviews of new books, an editorial discussing new developments in the life sciences, and a few notes and letters. The two semiannual cumulations abstract over 149,000 articles from 8,000 periodicals a year.* Appearing monthly, *BIOI* indexes additional research reports not in *BA* as well as symposia, reviews, bibliographies, book chapters, and selected government reports. Over 113,000 citations appear annually. A complete list of coverage, plus a description of how to search the indexes, is provided at the end of each cumulated index.

Both publications have the same kinds of index access, with reference numbers referring to the section with the bibliographic citation. These include:

1. The Author Index, which lists up to the first ten authors;
2. The *Biological Abstracts Subject Index in Context (BASIC)*, a computer-permuted KWIC index that uses the author's title augmented by significant words from the abstract and article. Foreign-language titles are translated into English. This type of index, without a controlled vocabulary, requires the user to prepare a list of as many synonyms as possible to search a subject thoroughly;
3. The Biosystematic Index, which allows a search to be made on a taxonomic category;

---

*A recent study in *BIOSIS Preview Memo* (vol. 1, no. 2, July 1979) notes that 78.8% of *Index Medicus* journals are included in *BA*. This, of course, refers to journal coverage but not necessarily to articles indexed.

4. The Concept Index (formerly Cross Index), which is an index by the subject concepts used in arranging the abstracts. While an abstract and its reference are listed under only one subject concept, it will be listed by reference number under all relevant concepts in this index;
5. The Generic Index, which provides access by Latin name to all organisms, except viruses, gleaned from authors' titles or keywords extracted from texts.

Thorough searching of these five indexes in either *BA* or *BIOI* is complex; however, BIOSIS provides helpful guides to their use in the introduction to *BA* and the *Guide to the Use of Biological Abstracts*. Even so, *BA* is, in most cases, easier to search online than manually.

Beginning in 1980, the *Bioresearch Index* will appear monthly under a new name, *Biological Abstracts/RRM (Reports, Reviews, and Meetings)*, and a new format, which will include a content summary for each reference, the language of the original article, and author's address. New book synopses will appear at the beginning of each issue as well.

4.15 *Chemical Abstracts*. Columbus, OH, Chemical Abstracts Service. Vol. 1– , 1907– .

Chemical Abstracts (CA) provides international coverage of the chemical literature from more than 14,000 scientific and technical journals, as well as conference proceedings, congresses and symposia, technical reports, dissertations, new books, announcements, and patents from twenty-six countries. Approximately one third of the literature is biochemical. Abstracts are arranged in eighty sections; sections 1–34 include biochemistry and organic chemistry, while sections 35–80 cover macromolecular chemistry, applied chemistry and chemical engineering, and physical and analytical chemistry. These broad section categories are issued in alternate weeks and cumulate into two volumes (twenty-six issues per volume) a year.

The indexes to *CA* are numerous and complex. Weekly indexes include:
1. an author index to authors, patentees, and patent assignees
2. an alphabetic keyword index to words and phrases from titles, abstracts, and texts
3. a patent index arranged numerically by country
4. a patent concordance that cross-references a patent either applied for or granted in different countries with the first reference in *CA* to the patent dealing with that invention.

Only the first reference to a given patent is abstracted. Volume indexes (semiannual) include the cumulated weekly numerical patent and patent concordances. Other volume indexes are newly constructed. These include an author index, general subject index, chemical substance index, formula index, and index to ring systems. Use of the general subject and substance volume indexes must be preceded by a study of the *Index Guide,* which lists entry points to the volume indexes published at the beginning of each collective period (five years) as well as indexing policies for the time covered. The current *Index Guide* appeared with the 9th Collective Index, 1972–76. Supplements to the *Index Guide* are published annually and are cumulative between collective periods. Use of the *Index Guide* is essential to proper subject and chemical subject searching of *CA,* due to the policy of controlled compound naming used by the Chemical Abstracts Service (CAS). In addition, a computer-based CAS Chemical Registry System assigns a unique "registry number" to a chemical substance, identifying it by a description of its structure, including its stereochemical characteristics. The *CA Registry Handbook* and its supplements provide access by registry numbers to *CA* index names and molecular formulas, thus providing entry points to the substance and formula indexes.

4.16 *Science Citation Index.* Philadelphia, PA, Institute for Scientific Information. 1961– .

The *Science Citation Index (SCI)* is an interdisciplinary scientific index, with 54% of its coverage being literature in the life sciences and clinical practice. Its uniqueness lies in the indexing approach it presents. In addition to an alphabetical author index, which includes a corporate index called the *Source Index* and a permuted keyword subject index called the *Permuterm Subject Index,* it provides a *Citation Index* listing the bibliographic references that are cited in current articles listed in the *Source Index.* The *Citation Index* also includes an anonymous citation index and a patent citation index. References are indexed from more than 2,600 journals and more than 1,400 symposia, monographic series, and multiauthored books. The index appears bimonthly (originally it was a quarterly publication) with annual and five-year cumulations. The latter makes retrospective searching relatively convenient.

The indexing of citations and their subsequent searching have definite advantages, but this approach also has some pitfalls. It is useful for locating current information on an obscure or new topic not easily defined by the controlled vocabulary of *Index Medicus* or even *Excerpta Medica*. It is also quite useful in updating references to an author's research or to the current uses of a specific technique or in identifying how well received or accepted an author has become. It can identify references to a topic in literature outside the primary discipline of the original author. On the other hand, cited references have their disadvantages. At present, citations are not checked for accuracy, and a miscited article may go undetected. The author's name may be cited inconsistently, using only one initial (either first or second) instead of two. For thoroughness, all possible permutations of an author's name should be checked in the index. In addition, the year, volume, or page numbers of an article may be miscited. Transposition of any of these numbers can easily occur.

The *Science Citation Index Guide and Journal Lists*, published annually, provides hints on citation searching and sample citations, as well as a list of journals indexed.

4.17 *Psychological Abstracts*. Lancaster, PA, American Psychological Association. Vol. 1– , 1927– .

Psychological Abstracts(PA) appears monthly with two volumes and volume indexes a year. More than 950 journals, technical reports, and monographs are abstracted from the world literature of psychology and its related disciplines. Dissertations from *Dissertation Abstracts International* are indexed but not abstracted.

The nonevaluative abstracts (some are signed) are arranged under sixteen major classified categories. Author and brief subject indexes are provided in each monthly issue, with an expanded and integrated subject index cumulated every six months.

Subject headings used in the subject indexes are assigned from the 4,000-word *Thesaurus of Psychological Index Terms* (2d ed., Washington, DC, American Psychological Association, 1977). In the monthly subject indexes, only subject headings and their cross-references used for citations in an issue will be listed. Three-year cumulated indexes are also available, and reference numbers to abstracts are consecutive within each volume. It is, therefore, important to note the volume and year when using these cumulative indexes.

A significant amount of clinically related material is abstracted in *PA*. It is especially useful for locating references to the psychological aspects of diseases and subsequent behavioral changes.

CURRENT AWARENESS SERVICES

Even with the aid of computers to compile and format the printed index and abstracting journals, there is a significant time lag between publication of a journal article and its appearance in an index or abstract. As a result, several rapid current awareness periodicals have been developed. The Institute for Scientific Information's (ISI) weekly *Current Contents* journals are the most notable. In the health sciences four are particularly popular:

4.18 *Current Contents: Agriculture, Biology and Environmental Sciences.* Philadelphia, PA, Institute for Scientific Information. Vol. 1– , 1970– .

4.19 *Current Contents: Social and Behavioral Sciences.* Philadelphia, PA, Institute for Scientific Information. Vol. 1– , 1969– .

4.20 *Current Contents: Clinical Practice.* Philadelphia, PA, Institute for Scientific Information. Vol. 1– , 1973– .

4.21 *Current Contents: Life Sciences.* Philadelphia, PA, Institute for Scientific Information. Vol. 1– , 1958– .

The *Current Contents* provides copies of the table of contents pages of current journals within weeks of their publication. (Not infrequently, *Current Contents* arrives in a library before the journal itself.) Author and keyword subject indexes refer to the *Current Contents* pages on which the reference appears. Also indicated is the beginning page number of the article in the table of contents for that journal, thus providing rapid access to the reference.

Excerpta Medica Foundation has recently entered the current awareness field with what it calls *Core Journals* in the fields of Clinical Neurology, Obstetrics and Gynecology, Ophthalmology, and Pediatrics. Combining the table of contents feature of *Current Contents* with abstracts from specialized subject journals, the *Core Journals* provide abstracts within six weeks of publication for articles in these specialties. The *Core Journals* are published monthly and provide no indexes. They appear to be designed for individual clinicians and researchers rather than for libraries.

There are many specialized indexes a library should consider carrying to satisfy the needs of its primary user population. This chapter has highlighted only the major ones in the health sciences. Consideration of new and additional indexes and abstracting journals should be weighed against a library's present holdings to determine if the new work(s) will be of significant value to add to the collection. Some of these considerations are timeliness of publication, provision of access to materials not indexed elsewhere, and provision of unique access approaches (i.e., report numbers).

REFERENCES

[1] see also Brodman, Estelle. *The Development of Medical Bibliography.* Chicago, IL, Medical Library Association, 1954. pp. 115–123.

[2] see also Kunz, J. Index Medicus, century of medical citation. *JAMA.* 241: 387–390, Jan. 26, 1979.

[3] see Austin, C. J. *MEDLARS 1963–1967,* Bethesda, MD, National Library of Medicine, 1968; and National Library of Medicine, *The Principles of MEDLARS.* Bethesda, MD, National Institutes of Health, 1970.

[4] see *Guide to Excerpta Medica Classification and Indexing System.* Amsterdam/Princeton, NJ, Excerpta Medica, 1978. pp. 82–83.

[5] *Oral Res. Absts.* 1:2, 1966.

READINGS

BioSciences Information Service. *Guide to the Indexes for Biological Abstracts and Bioresearch Index.* Philadelphia, PA, Biosciences Information Service of Biological Abstracts, 1972. (new ed. in press)

CAS printed access tools, a workbook. Washington, DC, American Chemical Society, 1976.

King, Michael M., and King, Linda S. *Guide to Searching the Biological Literature.* Boca Raton, FL, Science Media, a division of J. Husey Association, 1978. (slides/audiotape)

Science Citation Index Guide and Journal Lists. Philadelphia, PA, Institute for Scientific Information. Annual.

CHAPTER 5

Computerized
Data Bases

JO ANNE BOORKMAN

We are moving rather rapidly and quite inevitably toward a paperless society. Advances in computer science and in communications technology allow us to conceive of a global system in which reports of research and development activities are composed, published, disseminated, and used in a completely electronic mode.[1]

For health sciences libraries, the advent of the use of computers in retrieving references to the medical literature online began with the successful implementation of the National Library of Medicine's AIM-TWX (*Abridged Index Medicus* via *TeletypeWriter EXchange*) project in the spring of 1971. Developing from this project, MEDLINE (*MEDLARS*onLINE*), containing citations from the *Index Medicus, Index to Dental Literature,* and *International Nursing Index,* became available online in the fall of 1971.[2] Today there are more than 200 bibliographic data bases that have their counterparts in printed indexes and abstracts.

The computer technology that makes it possible for indexing and abstracting services to facilitate access to the rapidly growing periodical literature also makes it possible to manipulate the bibliographic information in a variety of ways. As a result, the data files can be used to extract citations for individualized demand bibliographies on a variety of topics.

Four major vendors†—SDC Search Service ORBIT (System Development Corporation), Lockheed/DIALOG, Bibliographic Retrieval

---

*MEDical Literature Analysis and Retrieval System.

†A data base vendor is a company that markets access to a number of different data bases acquired from data base producers.

Service (BRS), and the National Library of Medicine (NLM)—provide access to the majority of online bibliographic data bases used by health sciences libraries in the United States.[3] Each vendor provides detailed users' manuals (see Appendix 1) on how to search its system as well as specific information about searching the various data bases (see Appendix 2). In addition, some of the data base producers[†] have provided manuals describing their indexing policies and special features of the unit record.[‡] These manuals are essential reading for anyone actually searching the data bases; because this material is detailed and varies from data base to data base, there will be no attempt to cover it here.

According to a recent survey by Werner,[4] the majority of health sciences libraries provide online bibliographic searches through the reference department. In smaller institutions the entire staff provides the service. This chapter will, therefore, discuss the most widely used data bases in the health sciences as reference tools. Features of each will be discussed as they relate to their function in reference and as they complement the printed reference collection.

Whether or not the user should be present while the search is being processed by the librarian is a matter of considerable discussion. A survey of actual practice reveals that the majority of searches are processed by librarians without the end user present, and only rarely is the user allowed to run the search with or without assistance.[5] It is therefore essential that the librarian/searcher conduct a thorough reference interview to ascertain the full needs of the user.[6]

Often an individual will come to the library for a computer search when the information needed can be found readily by using more traditional reference tools. The user may also request a specific data base, such as MEDLINE, when other data bases may be better suited to the request or should be considered in addition to MEDLINE. Proper interviewing can suggest the appropriate solution to the user's need and save the librarian and user both time and money.[*]

In the reference interview the librarian must ascertain the purpose of the search to tailor it to the user's needs. A search to find references for a clinical care rounds presentation can and should be handled

---

†A data base producer is the organization that actually develops the content of the data base, e.g., Chemical Abstracts Service; NLM is both a data base producer (MEDLINE, TOXLINE) and a vendor.

‡*Unit record* is defined as all the bibliographic and descriptive components used to describe an entry in the data base: author(s), title, journal, keywords, page numbers, etc.

*Most health sciences libraries charge a fee to cover at least telephone communication and paper costs of the service.

differently from a search for a dissertation topic, grant proposal, research project, or term paper. The clinician may be satisfied with a
few recent citations on the topic, whereas the researcher and doctoral
candidate will prefer to have an exhaustive search processed over
more than one data base.[7] Cogswell points out that this individualized
service is not generally found with more traditional manual literature
search services. As a result, the service has led to an increased awareness by the user of the complexity of information retrieval and the
high degree of specialization and knowledge required of reference
librarians.[8]

A primary advantage to using a bibliographic data base versus its
printed counterpart is the flexibility possible in accessing the various
elements* of the unit record. While printed indexing and abstracting
services provide a variety of separate access points—author index,
subject index, report number index, etc.—the computerized unit record can be accessed simultaneously by requesting one or more of
these elements using Boolean logic.

Most often in bibliographic searching a combination of subjects is
requested, which is accomplished by using the logical "and." For
articles on nutrition in diabetes mellitus, for example, a search can
logically be constructed to request those unit records that have both
nutrition *and* diabetes mellitus keywords/subject descriptors. In the
following Venn diagram, the intersection of the two circles represents
those citations that fulfill the logical statement:

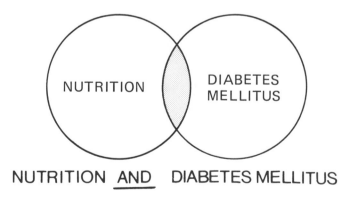

NUTRITION **AND** DIABETES MELLITUS

---

*An element here is defined as any single component of the bibliographic unit record—author(s),
keyword(s)/subject descriptors, journal title, year, etc.

The "and" logic allows for any number of combinations of the searchable elements of the unit record. The elements that can be searched in this way will vary from data base to data base and should be ascertained for each data base before running any search.

Two other logical connectors are used in searching. These are the logical "or" and the "not." "Or" logic is fairly straightforward. Articles on nutrition or nutrition disorders would look like the following Venn diagrams in which the shaded areas are what is wanted.*

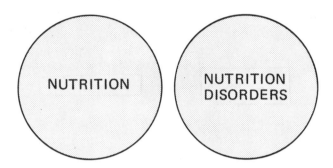

NUTRITION OR NUTRITION DISORDERS

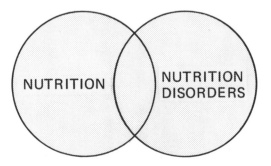

---

*Both Venn diagrams represent possible situations. In the first there are no unit records that have both topics as subjects. The second diagram shows an overlap where some of the records have both topics. This second diagram would, in all likelihood, be more valid with this example.

"Not" logic would look like this:

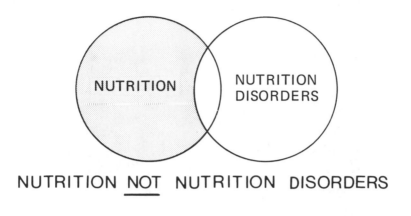

NUTRITION <u>NOT</u> NUTRITION DISORDERS

   The shaded areas again represent what is wanted, and the inter-section of those records mentioning both nutrition and nutrition disorders would be excluded. The "not" logic should be used with caution, however, because it can exclude desired citations if they are indexed with both concepts.

   As illustration, this topic could be searched in the *Index Medicus* using its controlled vocabulary *Medical Subject Headings (MeSH)* for appropriate subject terms (see figure 5–1). To search the topic thoroughly in the printed *Index Medicus*, references under each subject heading in the nutrition concept would be scanned for diabetes mellitus in the title, and references under each diabetes mellitus term would be scanned for a nutrition term in the title. Such scanning would be a formidable task, and it would undoubtedly miss potentially relevant references that did not have nutrition or diabetes mellitus terms in their titles.

Figure 5–1. Some possible terms from *MeSH*

NUTRITION DISORDERS (C18.654)
NUTRITION DISORDERS
  DEFICIENCY DISEASES
    AVITAMINOSIS
      ASCORBIC ACID DEFICIENCY
        SCURVY
      VITAMIN A DEFICIENCY
      VITAMIN B DEFICIENCY
        CHOLINE DEFICIENCY
        FOLIC ACID DEFICIENCY
        PELLAGRA
        PYRIDOXINE DEFICIENCY
        THIAMINE DEFICIENCY
          BERIBERI
          WERNICKE'S
            ENCEPHALOPATHY
        VITAMIN B 12 DEFICIENCY
        ANEMIA, PERNICIOUS
      VITAMIN D DEFICIENCY
        OSTEOMALACIA
        RICKETS
      VITAMIN E DEFICIENCY
        STEATITIS
      VITAMIN K DEFICIENCY
    MAGNESIUM DEFICIENCY
    POTASSIUM DEFICIENCY
    PROTEIN DEFICIENCY
      PROTEIN-CALORIE
        DEFICIENCY
        MALNUTRITION
        KWASHIORKOR
  SWAYBACK
  OBESITY
  STARVATION

NUTRITION (G6.696)
NUTRITION
  CHILD NUTRITION
  DIET
    CALORIC INTAKE
    DIETARY FIBER
  INFANT NUTRITION
    BREAST FEEDING
    WEANING
  NUTRITIONAL REQUIREMENTS
  NUTRITIVE VALUE

DIABETES MELLITUS (C18.452.297)
DIABETES MELLITUS
  ACIDOSIS, DIABETIC
    KETOSIS, DIABETIC
  DIABETES MELLITUS,
    EXPERIMENTAL
  DIABETES MELLITUS, JUVENILE
  DIABETES MELLITUS, LIPOATROPHIC
  DIABETES ANGIOPATHIES
    DIABETIC RETINOPATHY
  DIABETIC COMA
    HYPERGLYCEMIC HYPEROSMOLAR
      NONKETOTIC COMA
  DIABETIC NEPHROPATHIES
  DIABETIC NEUROPATHIES
  PREDIABETIC STATE
  PREGNANCY IN DIABETES

Precoordinated term describing a "nutrition disorder" in diabetes

OBESITY IN DIABETES

To run a computer search on this topic is much simpler and does not rely on scanning titles. The MEDLINE data base, the online counterpart to *Index Medicus,* has been designed so that like-concept subject headings are grouped together in an hierarchical arrangement known as a *tree.* Each tree is given a common number that can be manipulated so that a single statement groups the terms in a concept— the logical "or" relationship. In MEDLINE this grouping is called an *explosion.* Another statement can be used to "and" the two concepts and select those references that have been indexed with both concepts. In the example (see figure 5–2), a group of nutrition terms is "anded" to a group of diabetes terms. All subject headings for the concepts are used, both major descriptors (print subject headings in *Index Medicus*) and minor descriptors.

When formulating a search strategy, all possible terms must be used to describe each concept, since the indexer has been instructed to use the most specific term available. It must be kept in mind that the searcher does not know exactly what terminology an author used in an article or which term the indexer decided was, in this case, the closest *MeSH* equivalent for that article. With natural language data

Figure 5-2. Example of MEDLINE search

HELLO FROM ELHILL 3
YOU ARE NOW CONNECTED TO THE MEDLINE FILE.

SS 1 /C?
USER:
EXP C18.452.297   (tree number for diabetes mellitus)

PROG:
SS (1) PSTG (5321)

SS 2 /C?
USER:
EXP C18.654   (tree number for nutrition disorders)

PROG: SS (2) PSTG (5745)

SS 3 /C?
USER:
EXP G6.696   (tree number for nutrition)

PROG:
SS (3) PSTG (5799)

SS 4 /C?
USER:
1 AND 2 OR 1 AND 3   (logical statement combining diabetes
PROG: terms *and* nutrition terms)
SS (4) PSTG (468)

SS 5 /C?
USER:
PRINT 1 AU,TI,SO,MH

PROG:
   AU – FRANZ M   (sample citation with *MeSH* indexing
   TI – NUTRITIONAL   (MH). Note: Terms with * indicate
        MANAGEMENT   subject headings where the reference
        IN DIABETES   will be found in the printed *Index*
   MH – ALCOHOL DRINKING   *Medicus*. Terms marked with + are
   MH – CALORIC INTAKE   terms from the sample search strategy
+MH – DIABETES   that retrieved this article. Other terms
        MELLITUS /   like "diabetic diet" and the
        *DIET THERAPY   subheading "diet therapy" should
   MH – *DIABETIC DIET   have been considered for a thorough
   MH – EXERTION   search on this topic.)
   MH – FEMALE
   MH – HUMAN
   MH – MALE
+MH – NUTRITIONAL
        REQUIREMENTS
   MH – NUTRITIONAL
        REQUIREMENTS
   MH – PREGNANCY
   SO – MINN MED 62 (1):41–5,
        JAN 79

SS 5 /C?
USER:
STOP

bases that rely on keywords from titles and abstracts, ascertaining all possible synonyms to describe a concept is even more important for a comprehensive search, since different authors will use different terms for the same concept.

In addition to the "and," "or," and "not" logic, refinements are possible in searching so that phrases like "failure to thrive" or "type II cells" can be searched. The mechanics of doing this type of searching vary among the vendors' programs, but all provide mechanisms for this more precise search strategy.

Manipulating the system is only the beginning; good searching requires a real understanding of how the data bases are constructed as well as the level of indexing provided by the data base producer.

The data bases primarily used in health sciences libraries contain bibliographic data and have their counterparts in printed indexes and abstracts. There are, however, a growing number of data bases that provide factual information (CHEMLINE, *Toxicology Data Base* [TDB], etc.) but do not always have printed counterparts. These will be discussed briefly.

NLM DATA BASES

5.1 MEDLINE. *MED*lars on*LINE*. Bethesda, MD, National Library of Medicine.

The National Library of Medicine's MEDLINE data base was one of the first online data bases to appear for general use and remains the primary data base used in health sciences libraries. Its printed counterparts include *Index Medicus, International Nursing Index,* and *Index to Dental Literature.* The currently available MEDLINE data base holds the most recent two to three years of references (approximately 600,000 citations); the earlier years back to 1966 are available in two- and three-year file groups called BACKFILES. MEDLINE covers references to over 2,500 journals as well as a small number of conference proceedings and chapters from multiauthored books. The scope of the MEDLINE file is broad and includes basic life sciences material as well as medicine and allied health. The coverage is international, with one-third to one-half the citations to non-English-language articles. The average citation is indexed with approximately twelve subject headings from *MeSH*: three to five of them are designated as the primary concepts discussed in the article. These primary subject descriptors are the subject headings under which the reference appears in the printed *Index Medicus* (or other index). However, all twelve are searchable on MEDLINE and include such frequently mentioned concepts as *age groups, gender, geographic areas, experimental animals,* and *humans.* These concepts are not generally listed in the printed *Index Medicus.* The searcher using MEDLINE, thus, can search not only major concepts of an article but also secondary concepts discussed in that article. The depth of indexing is one of the strong features of MEDLINE as a bibliographic source, because the title of an article alone need not be relied on to reveal its scope. Keyword/textword searching of specific terms from the titles and abstracts is possible as a way of refining a search on a very specific topic.

5.2 TOXLINE. *TOX*icology Literature on*LINE*. Bethesda, MD, National Library of Medicine.

5.3 CHEMLINE. *CHEM*ical Dictionary on*LINE*. Bethesda, MD, National Library of Medicine.

5.4 RTECS. *R*egistry of *T*oxic *E*ffects of *C*hemical *S*ubstances. Bethesda, MD, National Library of Medicine.

5.5 TDB. *T*oxicology *D*ata *B*ank. Bethesda, MD, National Library of Medicine.

The TOXLINE data base provides access to references in the toxicological literature—journal articles, monographs, dissertations, published proceedings, etc.—from bibliographic secondary sources and to toxicology research in progress from the Smithsonian Science Information Exchange (SSIE) files. The subfiles include references (some with abstracts) from: *Chemical Abstracts (CA)* 1965– , *Chemical-Biological Activities;* MEDLARS 1968– , *Toxicity Bibliography (TOXBIB); Biological Abstracts (BA)* 1972– , *Abstracts of Health Effects of Environmental Pollutants (HEEP); International Pharmaceutical Abstracts (IPA),* 1970– ; *Pesticide Abstracts (PESTAB),* 1966– ; Hayes file on pesticides, 1940–70; a teratology file (TERA), 1960–74; Environmental Mutagen Information Center (EMIC) file, 1960– , a Toxic Materials Information Center (TMIC) file, 1971–75; an Environmental Teratology Information Center (ETIC) file, 1950– ; and reports and research in progress from the monthly *Toxicology Research Project Directory (TRPD)* and the annual *Epidemiology Research Projects Directory (ERPD).* The current TOXLINE file covers material from 1974 to date; however, several of the TOXLINE subfiles are complete and contain material as far back as the 1950s. TOXBACK contains most references prior to 1974, principally 1965–74; however, the Hayes file on pesticides contains citations dating from the 1940s. The TERA and Hayes files are in TOXBACK only.

This file, unlike MEDLINE, is searched primarily with natural language terms (free text) from titles and abstracts. The use of synonyms is the primary search method, including right-hand truncation of rootwords, i.e., to retrieve terms beginning with "mutagen," a truncation symbol would follow the term to indicate that all possible suffixes are wanted. Thus, "mutagen" would retrieve

> mutagen
> mutagenicity
> mutagenic
> mutagens, etc.

Logically this would be the equivalent of "or"-ing these terms in a search statement. The CAS registry numbers can be used to search the *CA, BA, IPA, PESTAB,* EMIC, and ETIC portions of the file. All *MeSH* headings cannot be used directly; however, "uniterms" (single words) from the *MeSH* vocabulary are searchable in the *TOXBIB* subfile.

Citations retrieved include author, title, source journal, secondary source identifier (e.g. *CA, TOXBIB,* etc.), and abstracts. The file has not been edited for duplicates, so the same citation may be retrieved from more than one subfile.

CHEMLINE is a companion file to TOXLINE. As a chemical dictionary, CHEMLINE provides synonyms and CAS registry numbers that aid in developing a search strategy. As with all textword searching, a large number of synonyms must be used to search effectively for type of organism, age, or sex concepts.

CHEMLINE, in addition to its uses as a dictionary file for TOXLINE, RTECS, and TDB, can also be searched as a data file for chemical information, including molecular formula and structure. In health sciences libraries CHEMLINE is generally used in the preparation of a bibliographic search in TOXLINE or other free text data base rather than as a search for more technical chemical information.

In the health sciences library setting, the files used for data about chemicals are RTECS and TDB. The RTECS file is based on *Registry of Toxic Effects of Chemical Substances,* the publication by the National Institute for Occupational Safety and Health (NIOSH), which contains toxic dose information. Included are threshold limit values, recommended standards in air, and aquatic toxicity data. Searches can be conducted on such elements as: CAS registry numbers (when available), toxic dose terminology, parameters of toxicity studies (e.g., oral, intravenous, etc.), animal tested (e.g., chicken, rat, etc.), NIOSH assigned number, or type of substance (pesticide, herbicide, etc.). The records contain actual numerical data with references to where the data were obtained. While the file has grown to more than 36,800 substances, it is still a relatively small data base.

The TDB file, containing approximately 2,500 compounds, became available in October 1978. Inclusion in this file has been limited to those substances with known or potential toxicity to which large populations have been exposed, and records are given full peer review before inclusion. More than half (1,500) of the compounds have full records, including chemical, toxicological, and usage properties. The remaining 1,000 compounds are still in the evaluation stages, and their records include name, TDB number, CAS registry number, and data extraction status. All sixty data fields are searchable. This file is linked through CAS registry numbers to the CHEMLINE file, indicating in the CHEMLINE records those compounds in TDB. CHEMLINE can thus be used as an adjunct to this file as well as to TOXLINE.

> 5.6 CANCERLIT. *CANCER LIT*erature. (formerly CANCERLINE) Bethesda, MD, National Library of Medicine.
> 5.7 CANCERPROJ. *CANCER* Research *PROJ*ects. Bethesda, MD, National Library of Medicine.
> 5.8 CLINPROT. *CLIN*ical *PROT*ocols. Bethesda, MD, National Library of Medicine.

CANCERLIT contains approximately 195,000 references from *Carcinogenesis Abstracts* 1963– , and *Cancer Therapy Abstracts* (formerly *Cancer Chemotherapy Abstracts*) 1967– , as well as selected symposia reports, monographs, and proceedings since 1977. Searching is done primarily using natural language terms from titles and abstracts. Abstracts in this file are lengthy and informative. As the source publications indicate, this file is most successful for searching topics related to carcinogenesis and cancer therapy, but not necessarily other cancer topics, which have been covered only since 1977.

Specific topics with no *MeSH* equivalent, like MOPP or DAFT, two combination chemotherapy acronyms, are more successfully searched on the CANCERLIT file than on MEDLINE. Conversely, topics that are broad or have many synonyms, e.g., embryonal and experimental tumors, may be more successfully searched on MEDLINE. In addition to the standard bibliographic information, citations include the abstracts and author address (useful for verifying a particular author with a common name and for obtaining reprint addresses).[9]

The CANCERPROJ file, sponsored by the National Cancer Institute (NCI), contains references to ongoing cancer research from the current year and preceding two years. This file contains descriptions provided by cancer researchers and collected by the Smithsonian Science Information Exchange (SSIE). Searching is primarily by use of natural language, although there is an hierarchically arranged list of subject terms available. Searches can also be run on institutions where the research is being conducted, principal investigator, and sponsoring organization.

CLINPROT, also sponsored by NCI, contains detailed information relating to ongoing clinical investigations of new anticancer agents and treatment techniques.

A wide variety of searches in the general area of cancer can be successfully run using the three specific cancer files and MEDLINE.

5.9   HEALTH PLANNING & ADMIN. *HEALTH PLANNING & ADMIN*istration. Bethesda, MD, National Library of Medicine.

5.10 BIOETHICSLINE. *BIOETHICS* on*LINE*. Bethesda, MD, National Library of Medicine.

5.11 EPILEPSYLINE. *EPILEPSY* on*LINE*. Bethesda, MD, National Library of Medicine.

5.12 HISTLINE. *HIST*ory of Medicine on*LINE*. Bethesda, MD, National Library of Medicine.

The HEALTH file, available since the fall of 1978, is produced in cooperation with the American Hospital Association and HEW's Health Resources Administration and contains approximately 130,000 references to literature in the fields of health planning and administration (organization, manpower, financing, etc.). The initial file contains references from MEDLINE, *Hospital Literature Index*, and selected journals emphasizing health care. References to books and technical reports will eventually be included. Searching primarily uses the *MeSH* vocabulary. The HEALTH file has the advantage over MEDLINE of covering references back to 1975 online, although there is a great deal of overlap between HEALTH and MEDLINE for the "current"

MEDLINE years. Citations are available with abstracts in some instances.

EPILEPSYLINE is sponsored by the National Institute of Neurological and Communicative Disorders and Stroke (NINCDS). The citations are obtained from *Excerpta Medica* and include abstracts. Subject searching is through textwords from titles and abstracts.

BIOETHICSLINE is a cross-disciplinary file of approximately 9,000 references to both print and nonprint material indexed since 1973 for the *Bibliography of Bioethics,* developed by the Center for Bioethics, Kennedy Institute of Ethics, Georgetown University. Included are references to journal and newspaper articles, books, court decisions, bills, state and federal statutes, and audiovisual materials. Searching is done using a combination of *MeSH,* terms from the Center for Bioethics' own thesaurus, or textwords in the title.

This data base provides the most interdisciplinary material of any of the NLM data bases, including references from the literature of law, religion, psychology, philosophy, and the popular media as well as the health sciences. References are all to English-language sources.

HISTLINE contains 40,000 references for the NLM *Bibliography of the History of Medicine.* Included are references to journal articles, monographs, and symposia in the history of medicine from 1970 to the present, with selected references back to 1964. The file is international in scope and is searched using a special vocabulary based on *MeSH.* The other NLM files—CATLINE (*CAT*alog on*LINE*), SERLINE (*SER*ials on*LINE*), and AVLINE (*A*udio*V*isuals on*LINE*)—are discussed in other chapters.

NON-NLM DATA BASES

5.13 BIOSIS Previews. Philadelphia, PA, Biosciences Information Service.

The BIOSIS Previews data base contains more than 8,000 references to literature in periodicals, monographs, dissertations, published proceedings, translation journals, nomenclature rules, and other sources indexed for *Biological Abstracts (BA)* and *Biological Abstracts/RRM* (formerly *Bioresearch Index—BIOI*). Each citation includes, in addition to the bibliographic reference, *BA* or *BA/RRM* abstract number, journal coden, subject descriptors provided by BIOSIS indexers, primary, secondary, and tertiary subject concept codes,* and biosystematic codes representing taxonomic groups of organisms discussed in the article. A language field was added in January 1978. (Prior to that time, limiting retrieval to specific languages was not possible.) Searching can be done using natural language words from the titles as well as keywords assigned by BIOSIS indexers, authors' names, and numerical codes for broad subject categories (concept codes) and taxonomic codes (biosystematic codes).

Searching the BIOSIS data base is much easier than searching the printed indexes in *BA* and *BA/RRM*. Use of the biosystematic and concept codes facilitates searching of broad topics and eliminates having to use numerous synonyms, but a search using the concept codes or the biosystematic codes in the printed indexes is laborious and awkward. Indexer-assigned keywords augment terms from titles with both common names of animals as well as genus and species names for animals not mentioned in the title of an article. Many words are segmented to add further flexibility to searching, e.g., Adreno cortical, neuro physiology, pseudo protein. The abstracts from *BA* citations, however, are not included in the data base, necessitating the use of the printed *Biological Abstracts* for that information.

5.14 CA Search. Columbus, OH, Chemical Abstracts Service.

CA Search provides online access to more than 14,000 journals, monographs, dissertations, conference reports, patents, technical reports, and reviews indexed for *Chemical Abstracts (CA)* from 1970 to the present. Keyword indexes from the biweekly issues of *CA* and CASIA (*CA Subject Index Alert*) controlled vocabulary of the volume indexes are included.

The unit record does not include an abstract but does include the *CA* abstract number, complete bibliographic information, journal coden, language, publication type, and keyword phrases from the biweekly issues of *CA* and the *CA* section where the citation appeared.

Searching is primarily by use of natural language terms from titles and keywords (and abbreviations in keywords) added by indexers; *CA* subject sections, authors' names, language, and type of publication are also searchable. (The CAS registry number is not a searchable element in all vendors' systems.) It should be kept in mind that the first five sections of *CA* are available in TOXLINE, including abstracts in that file.

*Concept codes are numerical codes used to index broad subject areas in biology, e.g., "Neoplasms" and "Neoplastic agents—diagnostic methods" as a concept could be searched using the concept code CC24001.

5.15 *EMBASE*. Excerpta Medica data *BASE*. Amsterdam/Princeton, NJ, Excerpta Medica.

EMBASE became available from Lockheed in 1978. The file includes references from all the sections of *Excerpta Medica*. References to articles from 4,500 journals (3,500 regularly indexed) comprise 95% of the data base, with references from monographs and dissertations comprising the other 5% of the file. The data base is limited to human medicine and the basic sciences related to that field. While there are some references to allied health, dentistry, nursing, psychology, and veterinary medicine in the data base, they are not specifically included, and specialty journals in these fields are not indexed.

Unit records in EMBASE contain the citation number (which does not correspond to an abstract number in the printed *EM*); the bibliographic citation; *Excerpta Medica* classification numbers, EMCLASS, for all the sections in which the citation was indexed, but not the section, if any, in which the citation was printed; the indexing terms from the MALIMET (*MAster LIsting of MEdical Indexing Terms*) thesaurus; natural language terms; EMTAGS, frequently mentioned concepts like "review articles," "fetus," "embryo," etc.;[10] and the abstract. In January 1979, EMBASE records began containing references to the printed journal. If a record is listed for more than one *EM* section, reference is made to the abstract number in the most relevant section for that citation.

Searching is done using a combination of free text and MALIMET terms, with author searching, EMCLASS, and EMTAG searching also possible. The MALIMET vocabulary has 180,000 preferred terms with 250,000 synonyms, which, when used, are automatically mapped to the preferred terms.

EMBASE represents the entire *Excerpta Medica* file, whereas the printed sections contain only 60% of the online file. This variation is in part due to the editorial policies of *Excerpta Medica*, which allow each section editor to determine whether citations included in that section are to be included in the printed journal section or remain available only online. That is, 40% of the records in the *Excerpta Medica* files are never listed in the printed sections and are only available online.

It remains to be seen how retrieval compares between EMBASE and MEDLINE in the area of human medicine. Judging from the protracted indexing procedures for EMBASE (8 weeks), MEDLINE will be more timely. Overlap of coverage will undoubtedly be significant.

5.16 PSYCHOLOGICAL ABSTRACTS. Lancaster, PA, American Psychological Association.

Corresponding to the printed version of *Psychological Abstracts* from 1967 on, the data base contains references to articles from more than 800 journals, as well as from monographs, dissertations, technical reports, and conference reports. Each unit record includes the *Psychological Abstracts* abstract number; bibliographic information, including author address; language; year of publication; subject descriptors from the *Thesaurus of Psychological Index Terms*; abstract; and subject index phrases from the volume and cumulative indexes of *Psychological Abstracts*.

A combination of searching thesaurus terms and natural language terms from titles and abstracts is most successful. Limiting searches to thesaurus terms can be restrictive with some topics, due in part to the fact that the thesaurus has been used only since 1973, and before that time only about 800 index terms were used. Two additional drawbacks of the thesaurus are imprecise definitions and only a single level of indexing that does not allow for depth or degree of importance in describing the contents of an article. Searching prior to 1973 is more successful, using free text terms. Language, publication type, year of publication, and author are also searchable fields. In addition, specific psychological tests are searchable. A search of this file often produces false drops or noise, which is difficult to weed out because of the multiple meaning of many terms in the psychological literature. A topic such as the psychological aspects of abortion could be searched appropriately on MEDLINE, EMBASE, and the *Psychological Abstracts* file.

5.17 SCISEARCH. Philadelphia, PA, Institute for Scientific Information.

SCISEARCH is a multidisciplinary data base indexing the literature of science and technology. Records correspond to the published *Science Citation Index (SCI)* with additional citations from the *Current Contents* series not included in *SCI*. The data base covers January 1974 to date and includes all significant references (articles, reports of meetings, letters, editorials, correction notices, etc.) from 3,700 scientific and technical journals. Subject coverage in the life and health sciences is roughly divided as follows: Life Sciences, 23%; Clinical Practice, 12%; and Agriculture, Biology, and Environmental Sciences,

11%. The remainder of the data base is composed of citations in the physical sciences and technology.

In addition to the bibliographic record, citations give information on language, author's address, and number of references, and include all cited references. Searching this file has some special capabilities due to the unique features of the file's records. Retrieval can be by natural language terms from the title and author address fields. In the *Citation Index* (comprising references from the bibliographies of *Source Index* citations), the following elements are directly searchable: name of first author, journal title, volume number, first page of the item, year of publication, and code for the type of publication. Note that the title of a cited article is not searchable, nor is it an element in the record. Thus, it cannot be printed.

The searchable fields in the *Source Index* include: names of all authors, addresses of all authors (where given), title in English, actual title (if not in English), journal title, volume and issue numbers, inclusive pagination of the item, year of publication, code for type of publication, number of references, and Institute for Scientific Information (ISI) journal issue accession number. Subject searching is strictly on natural language terms from the titles of source articles.

Citation Index searching can be valuable when it is known that relevant material on a topic will be scattered through more than one discipline or buried in the text of a seemingly nonrelevant paper, e.g., a specific method or technique with varied applications. Citations begin to appear from nine to twelve months after the original article appears in print, so very recent articles will not be useful for citation searching. The multidisciplinary subject coverage of this file is also a useful feature for some search topics. Another helpful feature of the file is the one- to three-week lag time between publication and entry onto the file.

Citation searching does have pitfalls along with its usefulness. For example, searching on a cited author's name, such as Harris TB, will: (1) retrieve all earlier papers written by Harris in any subject on any aspect of Harris' research that was cited, (2) retrieve papers because they cited Harris working in another field of research, (3) retrieve all papers citing earlier works by Harris TB, even though some were by Thomas B., some by Teresa B., and yet others by T. Bradford, (4) fail to retrieve articles that cited relevant papers by Harris when Harris was not the first author, and (5) fail to retrieve articles that cited relevant papers by Harris because only Harris' first initial was used in the reference or because the initials were inverted.

SDI SEARCHES

Selective Dissemination of Information (SDI) searches are available from BRS, Lockheed, and NLM for some of their files (the System Development Corporation [SDC] will soon provide SDI service); with this service search profiles are stored in the computer and automatically processed against each file update, usually on a monthly basis. For the files discussed in this chapter, BRS provides monthly SDI capabilities for BIOSIS, MEDLINE, *Psychological Abstracts*, and *CA search*; Lockheed provides monthly SDIs for BIOSIS and *Psychological Abstracts*, semimonthly updates for *CA* search, and variable updates for EMBASE; NLM provides SDI service for MEDLINE, TOXLINE, and CANCERLIT on a monthly basis. There are also commercial SDI services like the *Automatic Subject Citation Alert* (ASCA) service offered by the Institute for Scientific Information.

There are many other data bases that have relevance to the health sciences. The following sources provide more exhaustive lists of available data bases:

> Williams, M. E., and Rouse, S. H. *Computer-readable Bibliographic Databases: a Directory and Data Sourcebook.* Washington, DC, American Society for Information Science, 1979. (Looseleaf)
>
> "Data Bases Online." *Online Review.* 2:313–323, Dec., 1978.
>
> *Directory of Online Bibliographic Services, a list of commercially available databases.* Rockville, MD, Capitol Systems Group, Inc., 1978.

"Data Bases Online" has the potential for being the most timely reference; there are plans to make it a regularly updated feature in *Online Review.* It is in tabular form with information on files available from six on-line vendors (four U.S. and two British), giving subject coverage, vendor, beginning year online, and online charges for each file. The *Sourcebook* by Williams and Rouse is more comprehensive in its descriptions of each data base. *The Directory of Online Bibliographic Services* provides information similar to that in the "Data Bases Online" article.

Successful searching requires constant awareness of data base and vendor system changes. The vendors provide monthly newsletters to subscribers (see Appendix 1), which contain information on system changes and data base updates. In addition, the data base producers provide information on changes in their files, vocabularies, etc.

Other opportunities for keeping up to date on searching are workshops connected with library school continuing education programs, regional and local online users' groups, and programs at regional and national meetings of organizations such as the Medical Library Association.

Each library and user population will determine which files will be most useful for that library to offer, but the use of online data bases as a primary reference tool has become so essential that all provisions should be made to ensure that the reference staff maintains its expertise in as many search methods as possible.

APPENDIX 1

Online Searching Aids

Bibliographic Retrieval Services (BRS)

BRS System Reference Manual. Scotia, NY, Bibliographic Retrieval Services, Inc., 1979. (Looseleaf, various paging)

BRS Bulletin. Vol. 1– , 1977– .

Lockheed/DIALOG

A Brief Guide to DIALOG Searching. Palo Alto, CA, Lockheed Information Systems, Sep. 1976.

Guide to DIALOG Databases. Palo Alto, CA, Lockheed Information Systems. (Three looseleaf volumes, various paging) (Vol. 1, Aug. 1977, Files 1–25; Vol. II, Oct. 1977, Files 26–50; Vol. III, Oct. 1978, Files 51–75).

Chronolog, monthly newsletter of the DIALOG Information Retrieval Services. Vol. 1– , 1973– .

National Library of Medicine (NLM)

Online Services Reference Manual. MEDLARS Management Section. Bibliographic Services Division. National Library of Medicine, 1980. (Looseleaf, various paging with updates)

NLM Technical Bulletin. No. 1– , 1970– .

System Development Corporation (SDC)

SDC Search Service. *ORBIT User Manual.* Santa Monica, CA, System Development Corporation, Apr. 1975. (Two looseleaf volumes, various paging)

———. *ORBIT Quick-reference Guide.* Santa Monica, CA, System Development Corporation, 1978. (Looseleaf, unpaged)

———. *ORBIT News.* Vol. 1– , 1973– .

APPENDIX 2

Data Base Search Aids

MEDLINE

U.S. National Library of Medicine. *Medical Subject Headings, annotated alphabetic list (MeSH)*. Springfield, VA, National Technical Information Service (NTIS).

————. *Medical Subject Headings, Tree Structure*. Springfield, VA, NTIS. Annual.

————. *Permuted Medical Subject Headings*. Springfield, VA, NTIS. Annual.

————. *MEDLARS Indexing Manual*. Part I, Jul. 1976, Part II, Aug. 1977. Springfield, VA, NTIS.

NLM. *Online Services Reference Manual*. Chapter 7 MEDLINE/SDILINE/BACKFILES.

BRS System Reference Manual. MEDLARS.

TOXLINE/CHEMLINE

Medical Subject Headings. See under MEDLINE

CHEMLINE

Merck Index, an Encyclopedia of Chemicals and Drugs. 9th ed. Rahway, NJ, Merck & Co., 1976.

NLM. *Online Services Reference Manual*. Chapter 12. TOXLINE/TOXBACK; Chapter 13. CHEMLINE.

RTECS

NLM. *Online Service Reference Manual*. Chapter 14. RTECS.

Registry of Toxic Effects of Chemical Substances. Rockville, MD, National Institute of Environmental Safety and Health, 1977. 2 vols.

CHEMLINE

TDB

NLM. *Online Services Reference Manual*. Chapter 15. TDB.

Merck Index

CHEMLINE

CANCERLIT/CANCERPROJ/CLINPROT

NLM. *Online Services Reference Manual*. Chapter 16. CANCERLIT; Chapter 17. CANCERPROJ; Chapter 18. CLINPROT.

Technical Notes, MEDLARS Indexing Instructions. Supplement Tumor/KEY (a revision of the 1970 Tumor Manual) 1975.

Indexing terms and codes used in CANCERPROJ. Alphabetical Listing (Mar. 1977) (NLM).

CLINPROT Indexing Terms and Frequencies (May 1978) (NLM).

HEALTH PLANNING AND ADMINISTRATION

MeSH. See under MEDLINE

NLM. *Online Services Reference Manual*. Chapter 23. HEALTH

EPILEPSYLINE

NLM. *Online Services Reference Manual*. Chapter 19. EPILEPSY

BIOETHICSLINE

Bibliography of Bioethics. Thesaurus (located in the beginning of each volume).

NLM. *Online Services Reference Manual.* Chapter 21. BIOETHICS.

HISTLINE

Bibliography of the History of Medicine. No. 1– , 1964– . Bethesda, MD, National Library of Medicine (annual with 5-year cumulations).

NLM. *Online Services Reference Manual.* Chapter 22. HISTLINE.

EXCERPTA MEDICA (EMBASE)

Lockheed. *Guide to DIALOG Data Bases.* vol. III, Files 72, 73.

Excerpta Medica. *Guide to Excerpta Medica Classification and Indexing System.* Princeton, NJ, Excerpta Medica, 1978.

MALIMET: Master List of Medical Indexing Terms. Princeton, NJ. Excerpta Medica, 1978. (approximately 350 microfiche, includes EMTAGS and EMCLASS)

List of Journals Abstracted. Amsterdam, Excerpta Medica. Annual.

BIOSIS

BIOSIS Search Guide. BIOSIS Previews Edition, Philadelphia, PA, Bio-Sciences Information Service, 1979.

BRS System Reference Manual. BIOSIS Previews

Lockheed. *Guide to DIALOG Data Bases.* Vol. I, File 5. BIOSIS Previews; Vol. III File 55, BIOSIS Previews 69–71.

SDC Search Service. *ORBIT User Manual.* BIOSIS

PSYCHOLOGICAL ABSTRACTS

Thesaurus of Psychological Index Terms. 2nd ed. Washington, D.C. American Psychological Association, 1977.

Psychological Abstracts Information Service. *Users Reference Manual (PsychInfo Manual).* Washington, D.C., American Psychological Association, 1976 (looseleaf)

BRS System Reference Manual. Psychological Abstracts

Lockheed. *Guide to DIALOG Data Bases.* Vol. 1, File 11, Psychological Abstracts.

CA Search

CA Condensates Search Aid Package. *Keyword frequency list, key letter in context index, and frequency of words in phrases list.* (microfiche or microfilm)

BRS System Reference Manual. CA Condensates

Lockheed. *Guide to DIALOG Data Bases.* Vol. I, File 2/3/4, CA Condensates/Casia (CA Subject Index Alert); Vol. II, File 43, CA Patent Concordance.

Chemical Abstracts, Vol. 76. Introduction and Index Guide A–Z. Columbus, OH, Chemical Abstracts Service, 1973.

SCISEARCH

Institute for Scientific Information (ISI). *User Guide to Online Searching of SCISEARCH and SOCIAL SCISEARCH.* Philadelphia, PA, Institute for Scientific Information (197–).

APPENDIX 3

Online Professional Journals

Database; The Magazine of Database Reference and Review. Weston, CT, Online Inc. Vol. 1– , Sep. 1978– . Quarterly.

Online: The Magazine of Online Information Systems. Weston, CT, Online Inc. Vol. 1– , 1977– . Quarterly.

Online Review; The International Journal of Online & Teletext Information Systems. Oxford and NY, Learned Information. Vol. 1– , 1977– . Quarterly.

REFERENCES

[1] Lancaster, F. W. Whither libraries? or wither libraries. *Coll. Res. Lib.* 39: 356, Sep. 1978.

[2] McCarn, D. B. and Leiter, J. Online services in medicine and beyond. *Science.* 181: 318–324, Jul. 27, 1973.

[3] Werner, G. Use of online bibliographic retrieval services in health sciences libraries in the United States and Canada. *Bull. Med. Lib. Assoc.* 67: 5, Jan. 1979.

[4] *Ibid.*

[5] *Ibid.*

[6] see Somerville, A. N. The place of the reference interview in computer searching: the academic setting. *Online.* 1: 14–23, Oct. 1977.

[7] see Wanger, J. Multiple database use. *Online.* 1: 35–41, Jan. 1977.

[8] Cogswell, J. S. Online search services: implications for libraries and library users. *Coll. Res. Lib.* 39: 275–280, Jul. 1978.

[9] see Farmer, J., Guillaumin, B., and Sorrentino, S. CANCERLIT: a new look. *NLM Tech. Bull.* No. 109: 5–7, May 1978.

[10] see *Guide to Excerpta Medica Classification and Indexing System,* Amsterdam/Princeton, NJ, Excerpta Medica, 1978, pp. 82–83 (Appendix II, 2).

READINGS

Atherton, Pauline and Christian, Roger W. *Librarians and Online Services.* White Plains, NY, Knowledge Industry Publications, Inc., 1977.

Austin, Charles T. *MEDLARS 1963–1967.* Bethesda, MD, National Library of Medicine, 1968.

Christian, Roger. *The Electronic Library: Bibliographic Databases 1978–1979.* White Plains, NY, Knowledge Industry Publications, Inc., 1978.

Wanger, Judith, Cuadra, Carlos A., and Fishburn, Mary. *Impact of Online Reference Services: A Survey of Users, 1974–1975.* Santa Monica, CA, Systems Development Corporation, 1976.

Watson, Peter, ed. *Online Bibliographic Services—Where We Are, Where We're Going.* Chicago, IL, American Library Association, Reference and Adult Services Division, 1977.

CHAPTER 6

United States Government Documents and Technical Reports

FRED W. ROPER

U.S. GOVERNMENT DOCUMENTS

Most topics of interest to researchers and practitioners in the health sciences are treated to some degree somewhere in a government publication. As reference and information sources, government documents offer great potential for libraries in the health sciences. Unfortunately, United States government documents have traditionally carried a reputation of being hard to deal with, and as a result they are often underutilized. The difficulty of use derives from a lack of understanding of how our government is organized and of the specialized reference and bibliographic tools necessary for efficient utilization of the documents.

Government documents are those materials that have been issued by the authority of a government, whether or not the government has borne the expense of printing the publications. They appear in a variety of formats, from print to nonprint. Although the major supplier of United States government documents is the Government Printing Office (GPO), there are many other printing offices connected with the various government agencies. Not even the majority of the publications are printed at the GPO; however, the GPO serves as the major distribution source for publications coming from the various agencies. The National Technical Information Service (NTIS) (discussed later in this chapter in connection with the technical report literature) is the other major United States government distribution center for government publications

Government publications may be divided into three groups, roughly corresponding to the three branches of government. *Congressional* publications are those that relate to the work or proceedings of Congress, printed by the order of or for the use of either the Senate or the House of Representatives. The various court decisions published by the United States make up the bulk of the *judicial* publications. The *executive* publications are those published by the departments of the executive branch of the government or by the independent agencies in that branch.

Those libraries that have qualified for and requested depository library status may select the categories of publications most appropriate for their collections. Academic health sciences libraries are often associated with institutions whose main libraries have depository status, and they may receive the depository materials in the health sciences on that basis. Libraries that do not have depository status will have to select and acquire government publications from the GPO or other distribution outlets.

The frequent changes that take place in government organization constitute a major problem in dealing with government publications. As agencies are abolished, created, or merged, their publications may also change. Organizational changes result in variations in bibliographic entry, with difficulties thus experienced by the librarian in locating the publications in appropriate catalogs and indexes. The secret of successful reference use of government publications lies largely in keeping up with organizational changes and in mastering the various indexes and catalogs in which they are listed.

6.1 *Monthly Catalog of United States Government Publications.* Washington, DC, U.S. Government Printing Office. 1895– . Monthly; semiannual and annual cumulative indexes.

The primary bibliography of United States government publications is the *Monthly Catalog of United States Government Publications,* which has been issued by the Superintendent of Documents since 1895. Prior to 1940 it was not the primary index of documents; this distinction was held by the *Document Catalog,* which ceased publication in 1940. Since that time, the *Monthly Catalog* has become increasingly more comprehensive, and in recent years improved indexes have made the tool easier to use.

In 1974 the Library Division of the Superintendent of Documents' Office joined OCLC's online cataloging network, converted to the MARC format, and began cataloging according to Anglo-American Cataloging Rules (AACR). These changes resulted in a new format for the *Monthly Catalog* in 1976, and it has been a considerably improved source since that time.

The basic arrangement of the entries is by Superintendent of Documents Classification Scheme. Because of the interdependence of the scheme with the organization of the federal government, this arrangement is basically by agency. Author, title, subject, and series/report indexes provide additional access to the documents that have been included. Cumulative indexes are published semiannually and annually.

The current issues of the *Monthly Catalog* serve both as a catalog of documents coming to the attention of the Superintendent of Documents and as an acquisitions source. Prices are given for those documents that are for sale, and they may be ordered from GPO or from one of the other distribution sources indicated. The actual prices may not be the ones printed in the *Monthly Catalog* because of changes.

In addition to the general listing of government documents contained in the *Monthly Catalog,* individual agencies and departments may publish their own bibliographies and catalogs, and these should be consulted for specific items published by a unit.

6.2 *MEDOC: A Computerized Index to U.S. Government Documents in the Medical and Health Sciences.* Salt Lake City, UT, Eccles Health Sciences Library, University of Utah. 1974– . Quarterly; each issue cumulates; annual cumulation.

MEDOC is a computerized index to United States government publications that are considered to be of importance to health sciences libraries. It is prepared by the staff of the Spencer S. Eccles Health Sciences Library at the University of Utah, a depository library, and reflects the holdings of that library's documents collection. The index is online through Bibliographic Retrieval Services (BRS).

The basic arrangement of MEDOC is by the Superintendent of Documents Classification Scheme, and there are title, subject, and series indexes. Subjects are from *Medical Subject Headings (MeSH)* of the National Library of Medicine. MEDOC is published quarterly, with the final issue serving as a cumulation for the entire year.

TECHNICAL REPORTS

Technical reports constitute a group of materials that the health sciences librarian usually uses less frequently than other types. A special group of bibliographic sources maintains bibliographic control in the area, and it is necessary to become familiar with these materials if one is to use the reports effectively. Reports are not easy to use, they are not easy to locate, and there may be difficulty in some instances with their proper identification. However, a knowledge of the proper bibliographic sources and of the centers that are primary acquisition and distribution agencies for technical reports will increase the librarian's effectiveness in dealing with them.

The increased availability of technical reports through distribution centers and improved photocopying methods gives them the potential for greater use in research in the health sciences. Since World War II, technical reports, like other types of materials in the sciences, have been used more and more as a vehicle of communication. In the early period of extensive use, the technical report was considered only one step in the process of publication. It was assumed that a journal article or chapter in a monograph would result from the technical report. The technical report is now more often considered the final step in the publication process although portions of many of the reports still appear eventually in the more formal literature. Their more frequent citation in bibliographies and reading lists of all kinds is evidence of their increasing use, which places more pressure on the librarian to verify and locate the cited reports.

In general, a technical report either gives progress of an investigation currently being carried out or indicates the results of a completed investigation. The duration of the research project will determine the necessity for ongoing progress reports or one final report that covers all stages of the investigation. The report normally is prepared for the agency for whom the work has been carried out.

Quality of the content of technical reports tends to vary widely. Usually there is little if any quality control present in the form of refereeing. Material submitted to a journal, for example, undergoes much closer scrutiny than that in technical reports. However, the lack of restrictions on length and amount of material that can be included means that the researcher using a technical report has the potential for obtaining considerably more detail than would be present in a journal article.

Tallman has characterized technical reports in the following manner:[1]

1. There are many titles being published from a great many different agencies and organizations. Although there are not many *distributing* agencies, there is still enough complexity and variance to cause confusion.

2. There is a great range of quality in both form and content of the reports, ranging "from poorly written, brief minor items of ephemeral value, to near print, well organized and comprehensive reports of relatively permanent value."

3. Distribution is often limited and may be based on an established need to have access to the material contained in the report.

4. The reports are not available from the usual book trade sources; they normally have to be obtained from special distribution centers.

5. Bibliographic control of technical reports has for the most part been confined to the specialized sources; the more conventional sources usually ignore them.

6. No union list exists of individual library holdings.

7. Handling is difficult once the reports are acquired because they may have multiple personal authors, they may have several different identification numbers assigned to them, and the format may require binding or reinforcement for library use.

8. In many instances, the data reports contain may be of great value to the public and may be the only source of information available on the topic.

In the United States the major collection and distribution centers for these reports are government agencies: National Technical Information Service (NTIS), National Aeronautics and Space Administration (NASA), Energy Research and Development Administration (ERDA), and Educational Resources Information Center (ERIC). The principal center in the United Kingdom is the British Library Lending Division (BLLD).

National Technical Information Service

Established in 1945 as the Publication Board in the U.S. Department of Commerce, the National Technical Information Service (NTIS) has successively been known as the Office of Technical Services, the Clearinghouse for Federal Scientific and Technical Information, and the National Technical Information Service. Although its scope has changed with its name changes, the center's basic purpose of being able to supply copies of unclassified government technical reports has remained. Today NTIS serves as the "central source for public sale of government-sponsored research and development reports and other analyses prepared by Federal agencies, their contractors and grantees."[2] A collection of more than one million titles is represented in the NTIS data base, and each is available for sale. From this data base are generated *Government Reports Announcements & Index* and *Weekly Government Abstracts*.

6.3 *Government Reports Announcements & Index*. Springfield, VA, National Technical Information Service. April 4, 1975– . Continues: *Government Reports Announcements* and *Government Reports Index*. Mar. 25, 1971–Mar. 21, 1975. Biweekly; *U.S. Government Research and Development Reports*. Jan. 5, 1965–Mar. 10, 1971. Biweekly; *U.S. Government Research and Development Reports Index*. 1968–Mar. 10, 1971. Biweekly, with quarterly and annual cumulations; *Government-wide Index to Federal Research & Development Reports*. 1965–67. Monthly, 1965–66; biweekly, 1966–67.

6.4 *Weekly Government Abstracts*. Springfield, VA, National Technical Information Service. 1973– . Weekly.

Government Reports Announcements & Index (GRA&I) is published every two weeks by NTIS and includes complete bibliographic information plus an abstract of titles newly added to the data base. The basic arrangement is by subject; those areas of particular interest to health sciences librarians are biological and medical sciences, agriculture, and behavioral and social sciences. Since the NTIS is the center for distribution of government reports, some of the entries may appear in bibliographic sources from other centers. Reference is made to the appropriate source if the entry has already appeared in another title.

Weekly Government Abstracts (WGA) consists of newsletters in twenty-six categories, including biomedical technology and human factors engineering, medicine and biology, environmental pollution and control, and agriculture and food. The abstracts in *WGA* are published soon after the report is acquired by NTIS, and the primary function of *WGA* is to serve as a current awareness service.

National Aeronautics and Space Administration

The Scientific and Technical Information Facility of NASA maintains a data base of more than one million references in the areas of aeronautics, space, and the supporting disciplines. Reports included in this data base are abstracted in the NASA publication, *Scientific and Technical Aerospace Reports*.

6.5 *Scientific and Technical Aerospace Reports.* Washington, DC, National Aeronautics and Space Administration. 1963– . Biweekly; semiannual and annual cumulative indexes.

Scientific and Technical Aerospace Reports (STAR) appears semimonthly and includes NASA, NASA contractor, and NASA grantee reports, plus other reports in the appropriate subject areas from both the governmental and private sectors. A companion journal, *International Aerospace Abstracts (IAA)*, announces journal, book, and conference literature.

Energy Research and Development Administration

Energy Research and Development Administration (ERDA), which formerly was the Atomic Energy Commission, collects and disseminates information on nuclear science and technology. Until June 30, 1976, ERDA published *Nuclear Science Abstracts*, which included technical reports in its coverage of the literature of nuclear science from all over the world.

6.6 *Energy Research Abstracts.* Oak Ridge, TN, U.S. Department of Energy, Technical Information Center. 1976– . Biweekly; semiannual and annual indexes.

Energy Research Abstracts (ERA), the successor to *Nuclear Science Abstracts*, provides coverage of materials relating to energy, including technical reports, which have been originated by ERDA, any of its components, and its contractors; it appears semimonthly, with semiannual and annual indexes. Technical reports from ERDA that have been included are available for sale through NTIS.

Educational Resources Information Center

The Educational Resources Information Center (ERIC) is composed of a series of sixteen clearinghouses throughout the United States, each specializing in a different aspect of education, with responsibility for collecting and abstracting reports and other nonjournal literature. The acquisitions of the various clearinghouses are reported in *Resources in Education.*

> 6.7 Educational Resources Information Center. *Resources in Education* (formerly *Research in Education*). Washington, DC, National Institute of Education. 1966– . Monthly.

The monthly abstract journal includes reports and other nonjournal literature acquired by each of the sixteen clearinghouses. Items included in *Resources in Education* are available both in hard copy and in microfiche.

British Library Lending Division

One of the three divisions of the British Library, the Lending Division (BLLD) is located at Boston Spa in Yorkshire. Among its extensive collections is a large report collection dating back to World War II. The BLLD currently attempts to receive as many British reports as possible and has extensive holdings from other countries.

> 6.8 *BLLD Announcement Bulletin.* Boston Spa, British Library Lending Division. 1975– . Monthly. Continues: *BLL Announcement Bulletin.* June 1973–December 1974. Monthly; *NLL Announcement Bulletin.* 1971–May 1973. Monthly; *British Research and Development Reports.* 1966–71. Monthly.

The *BLLD Announcement Bulletin* has since 1966 listed reports from government and industry in the United Kingdom. Bibliographic information is provided in the monthly list, but no abstracts are available for the entries. In addition to reports, translations and doctoral theses are also listed.

REFERENCES

[1]Tallman, Johanna. History and Importance of Technical Reports. *Sci-Tech News* 15: 46. Summer 1961.

[2]*Information Work with Unpublished Reports.* Boulder, CO, Westview Press, 1977. p. 61.

READINGS

U.S. Government Documents

Katz, William A. Government Documents. In: *Introduction to Reference Work, Volume I: Basic Information Sources.* 3d ed. New York, NY, McGraw-Hill, 1978. pp. 323–343.

Morehead, Joe. *Introduction to United States Public Documents.* 2d ed. Littleton, CO, Libraries Unlimited, 1978.

Taborsky, Theresa. *CE 52: Government Documents.* Chicago, IL, Medical Library Association, 1979.

Technical Reports

Grogan, Denis. Research Reports. In: *Science and Technology: An Introduction to the Literature.* 3d ed., rev. London, Clive Bingley, 1976. pp. 241–250.

Morehead, Joe. *Introduction to United States Public Documents.* 2d ed. Littleton, CO, Libraries Unlimited, 1978. pp. 98–129.

Information Work with Unpublished Reports. Boulder, CO, Westview Press, 1977. pp. 53–81.

CHAPTER 7

Conferences, Reviews, and Translations

FRED W. ROPER

CONFERENCES

Since World War II, increasingly greater reliance has been placed on meetings, conferences, and congresses as an important means of communication in the sciences. More and more importance has been given to the role of the meeting in the social sciences as well. This situation has been equally true in the health sciences, and in recent years, the numbers of such meetings have greatly increased.

These meetings are considered a major means for the exchange of information with colleagues and for the establishment of lines of professional communication. For the librarian, they pose several challenges. Patrons frequently wish to know what future meetings are planned, where, and when. If the meeting has been concluded, questions will deal with the availability of papers given or discussed. Two major types of reference materials are needed to provide the information posed by these types of queries: calendars or lists of meetings to be held, and bibliographies of the published proceedings of the meetings.

Calendars

Information on future meetings is available from a variety of sources. The minimum items that should be provided by these sources are the following: sponsoring organization, name or topic of the meeting, the inclusive dates, the location, and, if possible, the name and address of the contact for additional information.

7.1 *Journal of the American Medical Association.* Chicago, IL, American Medical Association. 1848– . Weekly.

7.2 *World Meetings: United States and Canada.* New York, NY, Macmillan Information. 1963– . Quarterly.

7.3 *World Meetings: Outside United States and Canada.* New York, NY, Macmillan Information. 1968– . Quarterly.

7.4 *World Meetings: Medicine.* New York, NY, Macmillan Information. 1978– . Quarterly.

7.5 *Scientific Meetings.* San Diego, CA, Scientific Meetings Publications. 1957– . Quarterly.

7.6 *International Congress Calendar.* Brussels, Union of International Associations, 1960– . Annual.

The *Journal of the American Medical Association (JAMA)* publishes reference directories in various issues on a variety of topics including information on forthcoming meetings both inside and outside the United States. These directories are published every other month in the February, April, June, August, October, and December issues. The section, "Meetings in the United States," appears in the first issue of the month, and "Foreign Meetings" is published in the second issue of the month. Meetings are announced up to a year in advance of the meeting date. Each entry includes enough information so that the interested participant will be able to write for more complete program information. Journals of other organizations and general medical periodicals should also be consulted for meeting information.

A number of publications give future meeting information for all the sciences, including the health sciences. Such publications are useful in health sciences libraries because physicians and researchers are likely to need information about meetings in other areas of the sciences as well.

Through two separate publications, the "World Meetings Information Center provides information on meetings of international, national, and regional interest in the sciences, applied sciences and engineering, social sciences, and professions" (Preface). *World Meetings: United States and Canada* and *World Meetings: Outside United States and Canada* represent the most comprehensive and detailed listings available of future meetings in the sciences. Both are monthly and contain information maintained in the World Meetings Data Base.

The entries, which are arranged by date, are supplied for a two-year period from the date of the monthly issue. In addition to the minimum expected information, a considerable amount of detail may be supplied, including restrictions on attendance, availability of papers, paper submission deadlines, and a brief description of technical sessions. As more information on a meeting becomes available, entries are updated in succeeding issues. Five indexes provide access to the main entries by keyword, location, date, sponsor, and deadline for submission of abstracts or papers.

World Meetings: Medicine brings together in one publication all the entries relating to medicine found in the two more general publications. The format is the same as that for the other two titles.

Another publication also concerned with future scientific meetings is *Scientific Meetings,* which is published quarterly. The information included is similar to that provided by *JAMA.* Fewer details on the content of the meetings are given than may be found in the publications from the World Meetings Information Center, and there is no geographical approach. Emphasis seems to be on the United States and Canada.

The Union of International Associations provides coverage of international meetings in all disciplines through its *International Congress Calendar.* The *Calendar,* which is slow in being published, is supplemented by *Transnational Associations,* which is published ten times per year. It provides "a chronological listing of international congresses, conferences, meetings, symposia sponsored or organized by international organizations or important national bodies . . ." (Preface). In addition, there is a geographical listing by continent, country, and city, which provides all the information included in the chronological listing. Indexes provide access by meeting topic and by international organization.

Although these tools have as their primary function the identification of future meetings, they are often used to establish that a meeting was scheduled to take place. In addition to these current tools, there are retrospective lists of meetings that have been held. These lists may include information about publications resulting from the meeting.

7.7   *Congresses: Tentative Chronological and Bibliographical Reference List of National and International Meetings of Physicians, Scientists and Experts.* Washington, DC, U.S. Government Printing Office, 1938. (*Index-Catalogue,* 4th series, 2d supplement)

7.8   Council for International Organizations of Medical Sciences. *Bibliography of International Congresses of Medical Sciences.* Springfield, IL, Charles C. Thomas, Publisher, 1958.

7.9   *International Congresses, 1681 to 1899, Full List*. Brussels, Union of International Associations, 1960. (Documents, no. 8; Publication no. 164)

7.10   *International Congresses, 1900 to 1919, Full List*. Brussels, Union of International Associations, 1964. (Publication no. 188)

A supplement to the *Index-Catalogue* in 1938, *Congresses: Tentative Chronological and Bibliographical Reference List of National and International Meetings of Physicians, Scientists and Experts* provides information on some 17,000 congresses for which information was available in the Army Medical Library. For some of the congresses, very little is available beyond the fact that the congress was held and the date. For others, there may be information as detailed as a listing of the individual sessions held, along with information about any resulting publications.

The list from the *Index-Catalogue* is broader in scope than the health sciences. Included are those congresses that are of peripheral interest to researchers in the health sciences as well as those that are in direct relationship. In 1958, another bibliography was published under the auspices of the Council for International Organizations of Medical Sciences, the *Bibliography of International Congresses of Medical Sciences*. This list of congresses includes only those directly related to the medical sciences and identifies 1,427 congresses in the field of medicine. The basic arrangement is by subject with a chronological listing under each subject.

The Union of International Associations has prepared two lists of international congresses covering all subject areas from 1681 to 1899 and from 1900 to 1919. Each provides a chronological approach, giving the name of the congress, its location, and the date. *International Congresses, 1900 to 1919, Full List* includes a subject index for both volumes.

Papers Presented at Meetings

Often the papers presented or discussed at meetings represent the latest and most up-to-date information available on a topic. For the librarian, there is the difficulty of identifying the presenter, the title of the paper, and whether or not the paper has been published.

Cruzat[1] has identified six major forms of presentation for the proceedings of meetings:

1. A multivolume work encompassing the total proceedings of a conference or meeting

2. A monograph or report with a specific title and editor

3. A supplement, special number, or entire issue of an established journal that is often one of the official publications of the society or agency that organized the meeting, or because of the subject content of an individual symposium or conference elects to publish it

4. Selected papers or abstracts published in a journal because it is the official organ or because of subject content

5. Reports of a meeting or conference in a journal that has a special section devoted to "congress or conference proceedings"

6. Dual publication as both an issue or part of a journal and as a monograph or report.

In addition, the individual papers may be submitted to appropriate journals for separate publication. These papers then will be included in the indexing and abstracting services that index the journals. A problem arises when the paper has been revised and published under another title.

Identification of proceedings is further complicated by the current practice of taping proceedings, which may be the only format in which they appear. These tapes are not likely to be included in the traditional bibliographic sources.

7.11 *Conference Papers Index.* Louisville, KY, Data Courier. 1973– . Monthly. (Formerly titled *Current Programs.*)

Conference Papers Index, published since 1973, provides a listing of all the papers presented at the meetings that have been included, whether or not the paper appeared in published format. The *Index* covers scientific meetings, including those in the health sciences, and is prepared mainly from programs or abstract publications of the conferences. Arrangement is topical, and six of the seventeen sections are of direct interest to researchers in the life sciences. If there are publications resulting from the meeting, this information is indicated where necessary, as is the name and address of the individual paper presenters. The *Index* is particularly useful in those instances where a preprint distributed either before or at the meeting is the only known publication of the paper. The information is available as an on-line data base through Lockheed Information Systems, System Development Corporation Search Service, and Bibliographic Retrieval Service.

CURRENT BIBLIOGRAPHIES OF PUBLISHED PROCEEDINGS

The published proceedings of meetings may include the full text of the papers presented, or they may include only abstracts. Some will include everything presented at the meeting; others will be selective. There are several bibliographic sources that list published proceedings on a regular basis, although most of the sources will cover all the sciences.

7.12 *Index to Scientific and Technical Proceedings.* Philadelphia, PA, Institute for Scientific Information. 1978– . Monthly; semiannual cumulation.

7.13 *Directory of Published Proceedings: Series SEMT—Science/ Engineering/Medicine/Technology.* Harrison, NY, InterDok Corp. 1965– . Monthly, ten times per year; annual cumulation. *Cumulated Index Supplement.* Harrison, NY, InterDok Corp. Quarterly; annual cumulative volume.

7.14 *Directory of Published Proceedings: Series PCE—Pollution Control/Ecology.* Harrison, NY, InterDok Corp. 1974– . Semiannual.

7.15 *Proceedings in Print.* Mattapan, MA, Special Libraries Association. 1964– . Five issues per year (bimonthly excluding October); annual cumulative index.

Index to Scientific and Technical Proceedings (ISTP) covers published proceedings in all the sciences. It is a publication of the Institute for Scientific Information (ISI) and draws upon the various data bases of ISI for materials to be included. According to the Introduction, approximately 30% of the materials included are in the life sciences. The proceedings are listed regardless of the format in which they appeared, so long as they contain complete papers; those proceedings that include both complete papers and abstracts will be included. Published on a monthly basis, *ISTP* represents one of the fastest means of access to the proceedings literature.

The main section provides complete bibliographic information on the publication. Included in the entry are the titles of papers, the authors, and the addresses of the first authors in case of multiple authorship. Subject approach is provided through the Category Index and the Permuterm Subject Index. The sponsors of the meetings are found in the Sponsor Index. The Author/Editor Index and the Corporate Index give access to the authors of papers, editors of the proceedings, and the corporate affiliations of individual authors. The listing of authors and titles of individual papers is unique to *ISTP*;

the other listings of proceedings currently being published do not include this feature.

InterDok Corporation is responsible for two listings of published proceedings in the sciences—*Directory of Published Proceedings: Series SEMT, Science/Engineering/Medicine/Technology;* and *Directory of Published Proceedings: Series PCE, Pollution Control/Ecology.* Each provides basic bibliographic information for proceedings that have been identified in the respective areas of responsibility. *Series SEMT* has been providing information on "preprints and published proceedings of congresses, conferences, symposia, meetings, seminars, and summer schools which have been held worldwide from 1964 to date" (Preface). The principal arrangement for the entries is chronological by date of meeting, with indexes by conference keywords, sponsors, titles, locations, and editors. *Series PCE* is prepared from the entries in *Series SEMT* and a companion publication for the social sciences and humanities, *Series SSH.*

Proceedings in Print is broader in scope than the titles discussed above: coverage is in all subject areas. Proceedings are separated into two groups, with one section giving coverage to those titles published within the past two years and the other listing retrospective titles. There is a single index, which covers all current and retrospective entries in the issue and includes "corporate authors, sponsoring agencies, editors and keywords, or subject headings, as found in the proceedings, all arranged in one alphabet" (Preface).

These current bibliographic sources for proceedings, because of the information they provide, serve as acquisitions sources. They also serve as an additional means of verifying that a particular conference did take place. Through their identification of publications resulting from the meetings, it is then possible either to acquire the proceedings or to use other sources to locate another library that may hold them.

7.16 *Index of Conference Proceedings Received.* Boston Spa, British Library Lending Division. No. 69, June 1973– . Monthly. (Continues the same title issued by the National Lending Library for Science and Technology.)

7.17 *BLL Conference Index, 1964–1973.* Boston Spa, British Library Lending Division, 1974.

One of the most comprehensive collections of conference proceedings in the world is located at the British Library Lending Division (BLLD), which has provided since 1964 a listing of proceedings published in many formats. The monthly publication is arranged alphabetically by subject keywords taken from the titles of the proceedings. Within each of the keywords there is a chronological listing of all the appropriate conferences and the published proceedings. The scope of the collection includes all subject areas. The *BLL Conference Index 1964–1973* is a cumulation of the proceedings acquired during the ten-year period.

In addition to these titles that are specifically concerned with proceedings of meetings, the librarian must consult indexing and abstracting services for periodical coverage of proceedings and individual papers given at meetings. Sources for monographs, such as the *National Library of Medicine Current Catalog* and the *National Union Catalog,* will provide coverage of separately published proceedings.

In January 1980, BioSciences Information Service (BIOSIS) plans to begin a new publication (the successor to *BioResearch Index*) designed to provide coverage to meetings as well as a variety of other types of publications: *Biological Abstracts/RRM (Reports/Reviews/Meetings).* This new publication will give increased access to nontraditional forms of the literature of the health sciences.

REVIEWS

In an era of interdisciplinary research that requires the synthesis of information from a variety of sources, the review of research in the health sciences is a vital form of scientific communication. Through this medium, the primary literature may be reduced to a state that begins to be more manageable. By bringing together information about previously published research, the review provides the researcher with an overview of work that has been carried out in a particular area. For the student, the review may serve as an introduction to the topic; for the practicing scientist, it may function as a guide to a field that is only of peripheral interest. The researcher in the field will find the review useful to identify items that previously may have been overlooked or to update knowledge.

The characteristics of the review vary considerably. Generally, the review cites a large number of references and is confined to examining literature already published rather than presenting new information. Often the title will include such identifiers as "review of," "progress in," "advances in," or "yearbook of."

The review generally is found in at least two different formats. One is the serial publication, which is devoted to review-type articles, e.g., *Annual Review of Medicine, Biological Reviews, Progress in Clinical Pathology,* and *Year Book of Surgery.* The other is in the form of individual articles found in the regular primary sources of information; books, periodicals, technical report literature, etc. A third format to which it is more difficult to gain access is the literature search which normally accompanies a research study.

Bibliographic control of reviews in the health sciences has generally been better than that in the other sciences, due in large part to the efforts of the National Library of Medicine. Other agencies have routinely included and identified review publications in indexing and abstracting activities.

> 7.18 *Bibliography of Medical Reviews.* Washington, DC, National Library of Medicine. 1955– . Annual, 1955–67; monthly, 1968– 77, separately and in *Index Medicus;* monthly, 1978– , solely in *Index Medicus.*

> 7.19 *Index to Scientific Reviews.* Philadelphia, PA, Institute for Scientific Information. 1974– . Semiannual; permanent annual edition.

These two publications have as their primary purpose the identification of reviews, the former dealing with the health sciences and the latter with all branches of science.

The *Bibliography of Medical Reviews* is an ongoing feature of *Index Medicus (IM).* Beginning in January of 1980, it consists of a subject section that follows the same format as *IM.* Authors continue to be listed in the general Author Section. *MeSH* headings are assigned to the reviews included in the subject section of *BMR.* The monthly issues of *BMR* cumulate in the *Cumulated Index Medicus (CIM).* The *BMR* first appeared in 1955 as an annual publication; a six-year cumulation in 1961 represents review articles from the 1955–59 *Current List of Medical Literature* and from the 1960 *Cumulated Index Medicus.* It continued as an annual publication through 1967; and since January 1968, it has been published as a part of the monthly *IM* with an annual cumulation in *CIM.* It was also published as a separate monthly publication from 1968 through 1977. Beginning in January 1978, *BMR* has appeared only as a part of *IM.*

Since 1974, the Institute for Scientific Information has published the *Index to Scientific Reviews (ISR)* to provide separate bibliographic coverage of the world's scientific review literature. A semiannual publication that draws on the data bases used to produce other ISI publications, *ISR* represents the most comprehensive coverage of the review literature of all the sciences. In addition to monographic review series and review journals, *ISR* includes review articles in the *Science Citation Index* data base.

The *ISR* serves both as a source of bibliographic information for the reviews currently being published and as a citation index to these articles. In addition to the Citation Index and the Source Index, *ISR* has the Patent Citation Index, the Corporate Index, and the Permuterm Subject Index.

> 7.20 *Biological Abstracts/RRM (Reports/Reviews/Meetings).* Philadelphia, PA, Biosciences Information Service. 1980– . Monthly; semiannual index.

BIOSIS has announced a new publication in 1980, the successor to its former publication, *BioResearch Index. Biological Abstracts/RRM* is designed to give coverage to the nontraditional forms of literature in the life sciences with particular attention to reports, reviews, and meetings. The monthly publication will contain citations to a wide variety of formats that are not normally found in indexing and abstracting services or have had limited coverage in the past.

In addition to the three tools that are designed especially for the bibliographic control of reviews, the various indexing and abstracting services include citations to reviews and in some instances provide an indicator that the item cited is a review. These materials should be consulted for citations to reviews.

TRANSLATIONS

The promotion and stimulation of scientific progress and development depend on effective communication among the world's scientists. Frequently this communication is hindered by the language barrier. Significant research results that have been published in a language unfamiliar to a scientist have limited value. This situation exists with the biomedical literature as well as with that of other subject areas.

The researcher who cannot read the language of a research article has several options available. On the informal level, the scientist may consult someone who could offer either a partial or complete translation of the item in question to determine if a formal translation is worthwhile. On the more formal level, there are three primary methods available: cover-to-cover translations, translations available from translation clearinghouses, or use of a translation agency or a freelance translator.

Dealing with the bibliographic control of translations is a relatively recent development. Prior to World War II, no centralized translation service existed in the United States; thus it was necessary for the scientist to read foreign-language articles in the original language or to secure translations for personal use. With more global awareness in the scientific community, there is the conviction that access to foreign scientific writing is a necessity. This conviction has been heightened since World War II and particularly since the launching of Sputnik by the USSR in 1957. Particular interest has developed in publications from Eastern Europe, the Soviet Union, and Japan and the People's Republic of China.

There is little likelihood that scientists will develop a significantly increased facility in languages; as a result, their dependence on translations is likely to continue and even to increase. Since cost is an important factor in the production of translations, there have been attempts to share the costs in various ways, usually through publication of the translations or through pooling them and providing bibliographic access to the pool.

Translation Centers
Translation centers serve as a central collecting point for translations that have been made for individuals and organizations. The translations are deposited with the center, and the center provides bibliographic access to them. Usually the center provides reference service as well.

UNITED STATES
In the United States there are two major translation centers: the National Translations Center (NTC), located at the John Crerar Library in Chicago, and the National Technical Information Service, which is a part of the U.S. Department of Commerce.

The National Translations Center (NTC) began after World War II as an effort of the Science-Technology Division of the Special Libraries Association. Members of the division collected translations and maintained a union catalog. In 1953 the NTC was formally organized at the John Crerar Library. It continued its association with the Special

Libraries Association until 1970, when it became a department of the John Crerar Library.

The NTC serves as a major resource for learning of the availability of English-language translations in the natural, physical, medical, and social sciences. It maintains a large collection of unpublished translation and provides access to the published literature. For those institutions and organizations that donate translations to the NTC, it is possible to obtain access to the NTC's translations on a weighted basis corresponding to the number of translations deposited, e.g., 1–20 translations deposited, free access on a one-to-one basis; 20–40 translations deposited, 40 free availability searches, etc.

7.21 *Translations Register-Index.* Chicago, IL, National Translations Center, John Crerar Library. 1967– . Monthly; semiannual cumulative index.

7.22 National Translations Center. *Consolidated Index of Translations into English.* New York, NY, Special Libraries Association, 1969.

The *Translations Register-Index,* published monthly since 1966, is the current bibliographic source for NTC's translations. The Register section announces new acquisitions of NTC according to subject categories. The Index section is comprised of two parts: the listing of journal citations and the listing of patent citations. Journals are listed alphabetically by title, followed by the year, volume, issue, and pages that are available in translation from one of the sources listed in the Directory of Sources. The Directory is a listing of those institutions from which copies of the materials listed in the Index section may be obtained. Patents are arranged by country, and the Directory of Sources is used to determine from which source the patent is available. The Index cumulates on a semiannual basis, and it includes the NTC acquisitions that have been announced in the Register section. All Canadian translations are reported to the *Register-Index.*

For information on translations available prior to 1966, the *Consolidated Index of Translations into English* should be consulted. The publication is a cumulation of previously published lists from the Library of Congress, the Special Libraries Association, the National Translations Center, and a number of specialized sources. The *Translations Register-Index* serves as a supplement to the *Consolidated Index.*

The NTC provides a collection and distribution point for nongovernmental translations, while the National Technical Information Service (NTIS) collects translations prepared for government agencies both in the United States and abroad. Access to the translations maintained by the NTIS is available through *Government Reports Announcements and Index* (see chapter 6).

UNITED KINGDOM

The British Library Lending Division (BLLD) is the largest depository of translations in the United Kingdom and one of the largest in the world. Besides collecting translations, the BLLD has actively promoted cover-to-cover translations of Russian periodicals.

> 7.23 *BLLD Announcement Bulletin.* Boston Spa, British Library Lending Division. 1975– . Monthly.

Serving as a reporting mechanism for both technical report literature and translations acquired by the BLLD, the *BLLD Announcement Bulletin* is a monthly listing of these acquisitions. All items are held by the BLLD, and photocopies may be obtained. A list of issuing organizations is included along with some general information about the availability of their publications.

INTERNATIONAL

The International Translations Centre, located at Delft in The Netherlands, functioned from 1961 until 1976 as the European Translations Centre. It was felt that the new name better reflects the scope of the organization: the centers previously described in the United States and the United Kingdom concentrate on translations from a foreign language into English; the International Translations Centre collects translations into all languages.

> 7.24 *World Transindex.* Delft, International Translations Centre. 1978– . Monthly.

In 1978 *World Transindex* succeeded *World Index of Scientific Translations and List of Translations Notified to the International Translation Centre, Transatom Bulletin,* and *Bulletin des Traductions.* It is a subject listing with author and source indexes. All subject areas and languages are included.

Cover-to-Cover Translations

These publications, usually serial in nature, may enter into the normal channels of bibliography and may be indexed as a matter of course in the major indexing and abstracting services. For the librarian, discovering the availability of a journal that is translated on a regular basis may be a problem. Aids that will be useful in determining whether or not particular journals are regularly translated include *Ulrich's International Periodicals Directory, New Serial Titles,* and *Chemical Abstracts Service Source Index.* When it has been determined that there is an ongoing translation of a journal, the next step is to find out which indexing and abstracting service includes the translated journal.

> 7.25 Himmelsbach, Carl J., and Brociner, Grace E. *A Guide to Scientific and Technical Journals in Translation.* 2d ed. New York, NY, Special Libraries Association, 1972.

The *Guide to Scientific and Technical Journals in Translation* is now in its second edition. It provides a listing of those journals that are completely or partially translated and indicates the source for obtaining them. In addition, there is a guide to which volumes have appeared in translation.

> 7.26 *Journals in Translation.* Boston Spa, British Library Lending Division; Delft, International Translations Centre. 1976– . Annual.

The International Translations Centre and the British Library Lending Division jointly publish a bibliography of periodicals that are completely or partially translated. Unlike the *Guide* by Himmelsbach and Brociner, *Journals in Translation* includes journals that are being translated into languages other than English. While the emphasis is on the sciences, the scope of this publication includes all subject areas.

Cover-to-cover translations of journals originally published in a foreign language represent a significant portion of the translation industry. Bishop and Pukteris[2] have given a detailed description of the situation with regard to the literature of the health sciences. They note the expense involved in the production and acquisition of the cover-to-cover translations.

REFERENCES

[1]Cruzat, Gwendolyn S. Keeping up with Biomedical Meetings. *RQ* 7: 12–20, Fall 1967.

[2]Bishop, David, and Pukteris, Sophie. English Translations of Biomedical Journal Literature: Availability and Control. *Bull. Med. Libr. Assoc.* 61: 24–28, Jan 1973.

READINGS

Conferences

Cruzat, Gwendolyn S. Keeping up with Biomedical Meetings. *RQ.* 7: 12–20, Fall 1967.

Grogan, Denis. Conference Proceedings. In: *Science and Technology: An Introduction to the Literature.* 3d ed., rev. London, Clive Bingley, 1976. pp. 226–240.

Mills, P. R. Characteristics of Published Conference Proceedings. *Jour. Doc.* 29: 36–50, March 1973.

Reviews

Grogan, Denis. Reviews of Progress. In: *Science and Technology: An Introduction to the Literature.* 3d ed., rev. London, Clive Bingley, 1976. pp. 213–225.

Manten, A. A. Scientific Review Literature. *Schol. Pub.* 5: 75–89, Oct 1973.

Virgo, Julie A. The Review Article: Its Characteristics and Problems. *Lib. Q.* 41: 275–291, Oct 1971.

Translations

Bishop, David, and Pukteris, Sophie. English Translations of Biomedical Journal Literature: Availability and Control. *Bull. Med. Lib. Assoc.* 61: 24–28, Jan 1973.

Chan, Graham K. L. The Foreign Language Barrier in Science and Technology. *Int. Lib. Rev.* 8: 317–325, June 1976.

Chillag, J. P. Translations and Their Guides. *NLL Rev.* 1: 46–53., Apr 1971.

Grogan, Denis. Translations. In: *Science and Technology: An Introduction to the Literature.* 3d ed., rev. London, Clive Bingley, 1976. pp. 283–293.

PART III

Information
Sources

CHAPTER 8

Terminology

TAYLOR PUTNEY

To use the literature of the health sciences effectively, a clear understanding is needed of terminology and the tools that present the terminology. As is the case with general reference work, a variety of terminology reference works are available to aid in meeting the various needs of the user: comprehensive dictionaries of the health sciences; specialized dictionaries, such as those for abbreviations and etymology; terminology texts, the very specialized subject dictionaries; tools that work backwards from the meaning to the desired term; foreign-language equivalents; and compilations of syndromes and eponyms.

GENERAL DICTIONARIES

An unabridged medical dictionary is first of all a record of the usage of medical terminology. In a world where new diseases, new operations, new procedures, new syndromes are constantly being discovered and named, it is necessary that dictionaries be updated often. At any given time a dictionary should reflect the terminology that is currently in use in the medical professions. There are three unabridged medical dictionaries that are extensively used in the United States.

8.1 *Blakiston's Gould Medical Dictionary.* 4th ed. New York, NY, McGraw-Hill, 1979.

8.2 *Dorland's Illustrated Medical Dictionary.* 25th ed. Philadelphia, PA, Saunders, 1974.

8.3 *Stedman's Medical Dictionary.* 23d ed. Baltimore, MD, Williams & Wilkins, 1976.

Dorland's is considered by many to be the "dean of medical dictionaries." Now in its twenty-fifth edition, completely revised by a panel of eighty-five consultants, it is comprehensive and authoritative, and it has been a standby for many years. In addition to more than 1,700 pages of definitions, Dorland's contains many special features, foremost of which is the section entitled "Fundamentals of Medical Etymology." This brief introduction to the formation of medical terms includes lists of the most used prefixes, suffixes, and root words. In addition to the usual dictionary-type illustrations, there are twenty-six tables and fifty-two plates, all of which appear in their strict alphabetical order. In an effort to avoid printing the same definition many times, the editors have made extensive use of "see" references for words that are synonyms. In addition, anatomical terms are defined only under their official names, with cross-references included from common names. A major feature of word arrangement is the use of subentries. In the same paragraph as a main entry, e.g., "tuberculosis," will be definitions of the variations of that main entry. Each subentry appears in boldface type in the body of the paragraph headed by the main entry. Words and abbreviations in the body of the work are alphabetized letter by letter.

Stedman's dictionary is very much like Dorland's and is becoming accepted by many as Dorland's equal in authority and content. The latest edition, the twenty-third, has been completely revised by thirty- six editors. A useful feature of Stedman's is the opening section describing how to use the dictionary, which includes guides to pronunciation, derivations, abbreviations, and spelling of medical terms. The alphabetizing of terms and the main entry/subentry arrangement are very similar to those of Dorland's, and Stedman's also makes frequent use of cross-references to avoid duplicating definitions. Furthermore, there are many "see" references referring the reader to related information. Anatomical terms, eponyms, and chemical, biochemical, and pharmacological terms are included as main entries. Stedman's is well illustrated and includes 109 tables throughout the text and 31 color plates grouped in the center of the dictionary. Stedman's also includes a guide to medical etymology, which contains lists of roots, prefixes, and combining forms. The contrasting type faces and styles of type make it easy both to locate and to read entries. Of particular interest are the ten appendixes, which provide a great deal of information not usually found in a dictionary. The first appendix is a list of all the subentries used in the text of the dictionary.

Each subentry is followed by main entries under which the subentry can be found. Among the other appendixes are a summary of blood groups, common Latin terms used in prescription writing, weights and measures, normal results of laboratory tests, chemical elements, and a glossary of abbreviations.

The third of the major unabridged dictionaries, Blakiston's was published in its fourth edition in 1979. Perhaps not so well known or appreciated as either Dorland's or Stedman's, it is nevertheless an important work. The major differences between it and the two dictionaries just discussed is in terms of format. Blakiston's contains no subentries, but rather alphabetizes all terms and their subparts letter by letter. Synonyms are defined by the preferred term, and the preferred term is defined in full. There are no illustrations, but there are plates of excellent quality grouped together in the middle of the text. Like the other unabridged dictionaries, Blakiston's includes a brief guide to medical etymology. Also, like Stedman's, Blakiston's includes a number of very useful appendixes.

Though the description of the three dictionaries has emphasized differences among them, they really are very similar in terms of size, authority, and comprehensiveness. No two editorial boards will arrive independently at a completely comprehensive list of medical terms. It is difficult for editors to decide which terms should be omitted because they are obsolete, imprecise, or no longer commonly used and which new terms should be included because they are now widely used. Therefore, each of the dictionaries contains definitions that the others exclude. The individual health care practitioner or student can only be guided by format, readability, and special features, but libraries should certainly have all three on their shelves. The special features of each are reason enough for this recommendation, but the fact that the three do not contain identical vocabularies further accentuates the need for all but perhaps the very smallest libraries to own all three.

8.4 *Butterworths Medical Dictionary.* 2d ed. London, Butterworths, 1978.

A comparable title to the preceding three is the second edition of Butterworths, one of the two British dictionaries included in the discussion of general medical dictionaries. It is similar to the three American dictionaries in terms of vocabulary and comprehensiveness. Emphasis will, of course, be on British usage.

Just as there are unabridged and abridged English-language dictionaries, there are both types of medical dictionaries. There are two abridged medical dictionaries of particular importance.

8.5 *Taber's Cyclopedic Medical Dictionary,* 12th ed. Philadelphia, PA, F. A. Davis, 1973.

8.6 *Black's Medical Dictionary.* 30th ed. New York, NY, Barnes and Noble, 1974.

The introduction to Taber's states that it is an abridged dictionary intended for all persons in any field of health care delivery. This dictionary includes all the standard features of an unabridged dictionary, but it defines fewer words. It provides much information not found in an unabridged dictionary, however. Definitions are given for each main entry and for each synonym. No subentries exist, but Taber's does give many "see" references to related terms. Some special features within the text of the dictionary are descriptions of various accidents and first-aid treatment; detailed discussions of diseases with their diagnosis, symptoms, prognosis, treatment, and nursing care procedures; and entries for many foods with their nutritional content. Some tables are included in the text, but most are in the appendixes. A unique feature of Taber's is the "interpreter," a list of questions and statements that might be used in a patient examination translated into five languages. In addition, there is a fact-finding index that lists terms in the text dealing with diagnosis, first aid, nursing procedures, and poisoning. Taber's includes a directory of poison control centers throughout the United States.

Taber's is a good dictionary for paramedical personnel and for others who need a medical dictionary, but who do not need the complexity and expense of one of the unabridged dictionaries.

The purpose of Black's dictionary is best described by the following quotation from its preface:

> . . . a partnership is necessary between doctor and patient. Such a partnership cannot succeed without mutual understanding, and on the part of the patient this involves some knowledge of the working of the body in health and in illness. To help in achieving this has always been the prime purpose of this Dictionary.

Black's is written for the layman who must have some basic knowledge of medicine to interact intelligently with the physician. It contains main entries in boldface type, usually followed by long articles on the subject, which include much more than a simple definition. Broad topics such as "Insects in relation to disease," "Injured, removal of," and "Drowning, recovery from," are discussed at length. "See" references are used throughout to link various topics, but there is still much duplication. For example, there is a discussion of the thyroid gland under "endocrine glands" as well as under the main entry. Because the format and style are designed to be easily accessible to the layman, Black's is distinctly different from any other dictionary discussed.

8.7 Roody, Peter, Forman, Robert, and Schweitzer, Howard. *Medical Abbreviations and Acronyms*. New York, NY, McGraw-Hill, 1977.

8.8 Steen, Edwin B. *Dictionary of Abbreviations in Medicine and the Related Sciences*. London, Baillière, Tindall, and Cassell, 1971.

8.9 Hughes, Harold K. *Dictionary of Abbreviations in Medicine and the Health Sciences*. Lexington, MA, Lexington, 1977.

As has been the case with society in general, the health sciences have proliferated the use of abbreviations and acronyms, causing a need for current and up-to-date definitions. A recurring problem is the multiple meanings associated with abbreviations or acronyms. Thus, PPV may stand for "positive-pressure ventilation" or "progressive pneumonia virus," and SD can be "standard deviation" or "systolic discharge."

Medical Abbreviations and Acronyms, published in 1977, attempts to standardize the usage in the various health sciences. To that end, the authors have compiled and cross-referenced more than 14,000 entries. No definitions are given—only the full entry for the term.

Although Steen's *Dictionary of Abbreviations . . .* has a similar goal, there is less overlapping between the two publications than might be expected. A comparison of the terms between LD and LH indicates a similar number of entries, with considerable differences in the actual terms displayed.

The Hughes book also follows the format of simply giving the abbreviation and the full entry. It includes a wide variety of types of abbreviations, including journal titles, and is a useful addition to the first two works mentioned because of the lack of overlap. There are so many abbreviations today, no one source can possibly list them all.

MEDICAL ETYMOLOGY

The etymology of medical vocabulary is important to anyone using medical terminology because it explains how words were formed. Because the medical vocabulary used today is based on Greek and Latin prefixes, roots, and suffixes, the definition of a medical word is a combination of the definitions of its prefix, root or roots, and suffix. If one knows the definitions of the word parts, one can define the word. The importance of this fact is demonstrated by the inclusion of a section on medical etymology in each of the major medical dictionaries discussed earlier.

8.10 Skinner, Henry Alan. *Origin of Medical Terms.* New York, NY, Hafner, 1970.

8.11 Jaeger, Edmund C., *A Sourcebook of Biological Names and Terms.* Springfield, IL, Thomas, 1955.

Skinner's book is a general reference work of medical terms directed particularly to the beginning medical student. It is strongest in the basic science vocabulary. The format of the book is readable, and references are made to books or articles introducing new terms. Skinner does explain some eponyms, but discourages their use. One slight drawback for Americans is that most spellings in the book are British.

Jaeger's *Sourcebook . . .* is more complex and covers a wider range of words, hence the word "biological" rather than "medical" in the title. The third edition presents a text and a supplement fully cross-referenced to the text. The opening section provides information about how words are formed, types of words, and abbreviations guide. Both the text and supplement are alphabetically arranged, and each entry defines the word parts and makes reference to the supplement if necessary. There are numerous examples given, and some geographical and personal names are included.

TERMINOLOGY TEXTS

There are many books available to teach the student or health professional the basics of medical terminology. These books employ various methods, and they are arranged in various formats. Most current terminology texts, however, have the same goal—to teach the student the basic word parts (roots, combining forms, prefixes, and suffixes) that are combined to form medical terms. It is not the purpose of this section to review and describe all the available works, but rather to describe two works that differ in their approach in order to show the range of choices for the student who wants a book to help in the learning of medical vocabulary.

8.12 Young, Clara, and Barger, James. *Learning Medical Terminology Step by Step*. 3d ed. St. Louis, MO, Mosby, 1975.

8.13 Smith, Genevieve L., and Davis, Phyllis. *Medical Terminology: A Programmed Text*. 3d ed. New York, NY, Wiley, 1976.

The Young and Barger book describes itself as a "text for training allied medical personnel in acquiring a medical vocabulary." Its emphasis is on learning roots and combining forms and analyzing parts of words to understand their meaning, with an entire chapter devoted to a glossary of combining forms, prefixes, suffixes, and lists of Greek and Latin verbal and adjectival derivatives. Most chapters begin with a description of the body organ system and its component parts, processes, and mechanisms. Anatomical illustrations supplement the material, and at the end of each chapter is a glossary of the relevant terminology for that chapter. Special features include a chapter on the terminology involved in medical laboratory tests, a chapter of abbreviations and symbols, and a chapter that includes samples of many types of hospital reports. These samples are designed to test knowledge of medical terminology by presenting terms in context and giving the student the opportunity to define them from the context.

In contrast, the Smith and Davis book is a programmed text designed to teach medical terminology through repetitive use of prefixes, suffixes, and combining forms. In more than 1,500 frames, the student repeatedly answers questions and fills in blanks with the proper prefix, suffix, root, combining form, or definition. The student who knows word parts will be able to begin to define unfamiliar words through their parts. The book is intended for individuals working in medical fields as well as those whose work brings them in contact with medical terms on a regular basis. Many anatomical illustrations are included; and the book could be adapted for classroom use because the frames are conveniently divided into sections appropriate for individual assignments. Review sheets are provided for student use, and there are even eight tests included. Special features include a glossary of word parts used in the text, with references to the frame in which each first appears, and a list of additional word parts that could not be covered in the text, but are fairly common. There is also a list of medical abbreviations.

A unique feature of the book is the series of eight audiotapes available to accompany the text. They are useful in that they provide another method to study the word parts, and they allow the student to hear the proper pronunciation of each word part. These audiotapes are available separately from the publisher.

The book has been used successfully in classes for allied health professionals and medical secretaries.

CONCEPT DICTIONARIES AND WORD FINDERS

Most dictionaries consist of alphabetical lists of words followed by definitions. This arrangement is adequate if one knows the word. Sometimes, however, one only knows a definition or concept, not the correct word. Obviously, in this case, a dictionary that uses words as the access point is useless, and an inverted dictionary or word finder is necessary.

8.14 Rigal, Waldo A. *Inverted Medical Dictionary.* Westport, CT, Technomic, 1976.

8.15 Willeford, George. *Medical Word Finder.* 2d ed. West Nyack, NY, Parker, 1976.

8.16 Schmidt, J. E. *Reversicon: A Medical Word Finder,* Springfield, IL, Thomas, 1958.

The Rigal and Schmidt books are alphabetical lists by definitions or keywords, which lead to the medical term that is defined by the concept the user has in mind. Both are arranged alphabetically, but the Rigal book attempts to group the definitions under certain key headings listed in the back of the book. The *Reversicon,* on the other hand, may list the same definition several times, once under each keyword of the definition. Both books can be useful to anyone who uses medical terms.

The Willeford book is somewhat different in that it attempts to serve as a quick reference dictionary for secretaries, transcriptionists, and medical records personnel. The book is divided into several sections. The main section is simply a list of medical terms divided by syllables and accented for pronunciation. The remaining sections include a phonetic list of words; lists of arteries, veins, syndromes, etc.; lists of abbreviations used in medical records and medical writing; lists of medical specialties; and a list of prefixes and suffixes.

SUBJECT DICTIONARIES

There are numerous dictionaries available that are smaller and more specialized than a general medical dictionary. They are limited in coverage, and each has features that set it apart from a general medical dictionary.

8.17 Gordon, Burgess L., and Barclay, William R. *Current Medical Information and Terminology.* 4th ed. Chicago, IL, American Medical Association, 1971.

8.18 Boucher, Carl O. *Current Clinical Dental Terminology.* 2d ed. St. Louis, MO, Mosby, 1974.

8.19 Miller, Benjamin R., and Keane, Claire B. *Encyclopedia and Dictionary of Medicine, Nursing, and Allied Health.* 2d ed. Philadelphia, PA, Saunders, 1978.

Current Medical Information and Terminology is directed at the individual who must organize medical syndromes and diseases in an orderly system. The alphabetical arrangement, including cross-references, eponyms, and synonyms, leads one to the preferred heading for a particular disease. The authors indicate that their system of classification is even suitable for computerization. Each preferred entry includes the term, its code number in the system, and other information, including synonyms, etiology, physical signs, laboratory data, and pathology. There is a keyword index that focuses on etiology, an index of diseases by body system, and a section of abbreviations. The book is excellent in that it shows how diseases can be categorized for retrieval or statistical purposes.

Dental terminology is often confusing because of the number of different specialties and subspecialties in dentistry. Relatively simple and straightforward, this book by Boucher attempts to define more than 10,000 terms from twenty-three areas of dental practice, distinguishing the differences in meanings of the same word for different specialists. The arrangement is alphabetical, and a pronunciation guide is provided in the appendix.

Miller and Keane serves as an excellent dictionary for anyone in any of the allied medical professions because it consists of the terminology most likely to be used by these professions. Though the title indicates the book is also an encyclopedia, most entries are simply definitions. Words are divided by syllables and marked for pronunciation, and there are good anatomical tables and plates. Like the major medical dictionaries, this dictionary has as one of its best features the appendixes, which include not only the usual weights and measures, but such useful information as pulmonary function values, 1974 daily dietary allowances, sources of patient education materials, laboratory reference values, and voluntary health and welfare agencies.

8.20   Henderson, I. F., and Henderson, W. D. *A Dictionary of Biological Terms*. 8th ed. by J. H. Kenneth. New York, NY, Van Nostrand, 1963.

8.21   Gray, Peter. *A Dictionary of the Biological Sciences*, New York, NY, Reinhold, 1967.

Because general medical dictionaries usually provide little coverage of the more general biological terminology that is directly related to the health sciences, dictionaries of biological terms are needed. The Henderson dictionary is a general alphabetical listing of biological words in all biological and basic medical sciences. A straightforward, uncomplicated, unadorned dictionary, it contains over 16,000 terms, and all Greek and Russian terms are transliterated. One drawback to the book is that British spelling is used. The Gray dictionary is more complicated in that the arrangement is alphabetical for major terms like taxa or chemical terms, but thesauric for descriptive terms that require an extended definition. Like the Henderson book, this dictionary is directed to the generalist. It includes some vernacular terms, several thousand word roots, some personal names, and taxa above ordinal rank. Latin and Greek words are anglicized whenever possible. There is also a bibliography of works consulted by the author.

FOREIGN LANGUAGE DICTIONARIES

8.22   *Elsevier's Medical Dictionary in Five Languages*. 2d rev. ed. New York, NY, Elsevier, 1975.

8.23   Lépine, Pierre, and Peacock, Philip R. *Dictionary (French-English, English-French) of Medical and Biological Terms*. Paris, Flammarion Médicine Sciences, 1974.

Often it is necessary to translate a medical term from one language to another, and there are many dictionaries available that translate words from another language into English or vice versa. Elsevier's dictionary combines four such dictionaries in one. The main section of the book is a table with the English term on the left and the French, Italian, Spanish, and German equivalents on the right. Each of the 20,000 entries has a unique number. The second section is a list of English-language synonyms with a reference back to the entry number of the defined term. The last four sections are, of course, alphabetical listings of terms in each of the other languages, referenced back to the entry number of the appropriate English word. This format, though often requiring the user to look in two or more places to get all the needed information, saves space and allows for the inclusion of four dictionaries in the space of one.

The dictionary by Lépine and Peacock is a good example of the usual two-language dictionaries mentioned earlier. It is very simple in format—two sections, one with English entries and their French translations, and one with French entries and English translations. One added feature of this dictionary is the fact that brief definitions of terms are given if there is no direct translation from one language to another. There is an abbreviations list and a group of conversion tables for temperatures and weights and measures. There are many dictionaries available that follow this format for English translation into almost any other language.

SYNDROMES, EPONYMS, AND QUOTATIONS

A syndrome is a constant pattern or grouping of abnormal signs or symptoms. Important to physicians because they are usually associated with diseases, some syndromes have descriptive names, and some are named after the individual who first described the syndrome to the medical world. These latter names are eponymic. Each of these books contains lists and various amounts of information about syndromes, but each is different from the others.

8.24 Magalini, Sergio. *Dictionary of Medical Syndromes.* Philadelphia, PA, Lippincott, 1971.

8.25 Durham, Robert H. *Encyclopedia of Medical Syndromes.* New York, NY, Hoeber, 1960.

8.26 Jablonski, Stanley. *Illustrated Dictionary of Eponymic Syndromes, Diseases, and their Synonyms.* Philadelphia, PA, Saunders, 1969.

The Magalini book is probably the most comprehensive in terms of information about each listed syndrome. Most, but usually not all, of the following information is listed briefly under each entry: name of syndrome, synonyms, signs, etiology, pathology, diagnostic proce- dures, therapy, prognosis, bibliography. The format is easily readable and designed for quick reference. Though the text is not cross-refer- enced, the index is fully cross-referenced to the major headings.

The Durham book is not so detailed as the Magalini book, but it is still useful because it contains syndromes the Magalini does not. It differs from the Magalini in that the syndromes are cross-referenced in the text and there is an index by classification (type or organ system). The Durham book also contains references to the literature that elaborate on or clarify the syndrome in question.

The Jablonski book lists syndromes and diseases named after peo- ple (eponyms). Illustrations are used where they are helpful in de- scribing the syndrome. A typical entry begins with the name of the person for whom the syndrome or condition is named, the eponym, its synonyms, the definition, and a bibliography, which is usually a reference to the original report of the syndrome or disease. Synonyms, too, are listed separately.

8.27 Strauss, Maurice B. *Familiar Medical Quotations*. Boston, MA, Little, Brown, 1968.

8.28 Kelly, Emerson Crosby. *Encyclopedia of Medical Sources*. Balti- more, MD, Williams & Wilkins, 1948.

Important statements have been made about medicine, disease, health care, and other health-related subjects by all types of people. Strauss has brought together more than 7,000 such quotations in his book. The quotations are arranged alphabetically by category, and then chronologically within categories. The index, an alphabetical listing of keywords from the quotations, gives general access to the quotations. The book is authoritative in that nearly all quotations have been verified. When a quotation could not be verified, a sec- ondary source is usually given. The book is a compendium of who said what in the health sciences.

The title of Kelly et al.'s work is somewhat misleading, as the book is a list of names and the medical discoveries attributed to those individuals. Included are anatomical points of reference, operations, tests, treatments, diseases, or important writings. Also given is the source of publication of the discovery. The book is fully cross-refer- enced, and more than 6,000 names are included. The index works backwards in that it lists the anatomical parts, tests, diseases, etc., and the names associated with those items.

CHAPTER 9

Handbooks
and
Manuals

FRED W. ROPER

Handbooks and manuals are of prime importance to the researcher in the health sciences. These publications are compendia of vast amounts of information on a variety of topics and are useful in answering the so-called "factual" question. Grogan states that "a library with no more than a sound collection of handbooks can answer 90 percent of quick-reference queries."[1] They generally contain factual information of a practical nature to assist the researcher or clinician in day-to-day work. In format, they range from the one-volume data book to multivolume compendia, which may be encyclopedic in nature. This chapter deals with three types of handbooks and manuals: data books, laboratory compendia, and handbooks relating to physiology, diagnosis, and classification.

DATA BOOKS

The purpose of data books is to present basic scientific information in a concise format. Tables, such as the properties of substances, mathematical data, boiling points, and toxicities, are often used in the presentation of the data, sometimes accompanied by text. Frequent revision is necessary to assure that the material presented is up to date. The key to successful use of the data book is an adequate and detailed index.

9.1 Altman, Philip, and Dittmer, Dorothy, eds. *Biology Data Book.* 3d ed. 3 vols. Bethesda, MD, Federation of American Societies for Experimental Biology, 1972–74.

9.2 ———. *Growth, Including Reproduction and Morphological Development*. Washington, DC, Federation of American Societies for Experimental Biology. 1962.

9.3 Altman, Philip, and Katz, Dorothy, eds. *Human Health and Disease*. Bethesda, MD, Federation of American Societies for Experimental Biology, 1977.

These important publications from the Federation of American Societies for Experimental Biology (FASEB) are based on contributions from a large number of research scientists.

The *Biology Data Book* is intended to serve as a basic reference in the field of biology. With broadened scope and coverage in the second edition, the revised publication has appeared as three volumes: Volume I, genetics and cytology, reproduction, development, and growth; Volume II, biological regulators and toxins, environment and survival, and parasitism; Volume III, nutrition, digestion and excretion, metabolism, respiration and circulation, and blood and other body fluids. Each volume is indexed independently. An important feature is the inclusion of references for the sources of the data. Coverage is restricted "to man and the more important laboratory, domestic, commercial, and field organisms"(Preface). Even so, many species are included.

Growth is an example of the specialized handbooks that have been produced under the auspices of FASEB. Similar in format to the *Biology Data Book,* it is a compendium that presents data on various aspects of normal growth. The most recent title in the series of biological handbooks is *Human Health and Disease.* The seven sections of the handbook present data in the form of 186 tables of quantitative and descriptive data. Contributors are identified, and the series continues to include citations to the literature.

9.4 Ciba-Geigy Limited. *Scientific Tables.* Edited by K. Diem and C. Lentner. 7th ed. Basle, Geigy, 1970.

Scientific Tables is intended "to provide doctors and biologists with basic data in a concise form. . . ." The seventh edition has increased coverage of the mathematical, physical, and chemical data and includes a new chapter on biochemistry. References to the sources of the data are a part of each presentation.

9.5 Weast, Robert C., ed. *Handbook of Chemistry and Physics.* 60th ed. Cleveland, OH, CRC Press, 1979.

9.6 *Composite Index for CRC Handbooks*. 2d ed. Cleveland, OH, CRC Press, 1977.

9.7 Fasman, Gerald D., ed. *Handbook of Biochemistry and Molecular Biology*. 3d ed. Cleveland, OH, CRC Press, 1976.

An important group of handbooks is published by the CRC Press. Numbering more than fifty titles, the series is intended to provide coverage of many subject areas in the sciences. Titles in the series range from broad areas such as chemistry and physics to specialized topics such as chemical laboratory science, laboratory safety, and applied optics. Many of the titles are multivolume.

The tremendous growth of scientific knowledge in the twentieth century has led to the expansion of titles since the first title, *Handbook of Chemistry and Physics*, appeared in 1913.

With the increase of available data and the ever-growing interdisciplinary nature of science, the CRC Handbook series has expanded to try to meet reference requirements of the newer disciplines through the development of comprehensive multivolume handbooks. The *Handbook of Biochemistry and Molecular Biology* effectively demonstrates this concept. The third edition is published in nine volumes, which cover proteins; nucleic acids; lipids, carbohydrates, and steroids; and physical and chemical data. Other titles in the series have expanded in the same manner.

To provide a master key to the material contained in the CRC handbooks, the *CRC Composite Index* has been published. Material included in several of the handbooks or in the individual volumes in a particular title may be of value to the researcher. This necessitates checking the index of each volume. To assist in the gathering of data that may be contained in the various titles, the *Index* alphabetically merges all individual volume indexes into the simple series index. The result is a two-part index that allows access by subject and by chemical substance. The volume and page number are given for each entry.

9.8 *Report of the Task Group on Reference Man*. Report No. 23, International Commission on Radiological Protection. New York, NY, Pergamon Press, 1977.

Although the report was prepared to assist in studies on the effects of radiation on man, the data that have been included cause it to have broad application. The compilers limited their attention to those characteristics of man "which are known to be important or which are likely to be significant for estimation of dose from sources of radiation within or outside the body. . . ." Even with this limitation, the book serves as an important complement to the handbooks discussed above.

LABORATORY COMPENDIA

These materials serve both an encyclopedia and a textbook function. They generally consist of essays relating to techniques, methodology, interpretation, and analysis used in diagnosis. Representative examples include:

9.9   Henry, John B., ed. *Todd-Sanford-Davidsohn Clinical Diagnosis and Management by Laboratory Methods.* 16th ed. Philadelphia, PA, Saunders, 1979.

9.10   Frankel, Sam, Reitman, Stanley, and Sonnenwirth, Alex. *Gradwohl's Clinical Laboratory Methods and Diagnosis.* 8th ed. St. Louis, MO, Mosby, 1979.

9.11   *Methods in Enzymology.* New York, NY, Academic Press. Vol. 1– . 1955.

Clinical Diagnosis and Management by Laboratory Methods, through a series of essays, has presented in six parts the following organization of the laboratory:

(1) Chemical pathology and clinical chemistry; (2) Medical microscopy and examination of other body fluids; (3) Hematology and coagulation; (4) Immunology and immunopathology; (5) Medical microbiology; (6) Administration of the clinical laboratory.

There are sixty-three chapters, which explore the development of laboratory medicine and its application to medical care. The sixteenth edition "embraces a complete as well as thorough revision that is consistent with the new title of this text, as well as the role of the laboratory through its professional staff in not only translating this information into patient care, but also facilitating and amplifying the effectiveness of medical care delivery through sophisticated medical technology coupled with medical and scientific skills and knowledge" (Preface).

The goals for the eighth edition of *Gradwohl's Clinical Laboratory Methods and Diagnosis* are very close to those of the previous title— that is, to serve as a reference source, textbook, and laboratory manual. Differences occur, however, in organization and emphasis.

Both titles are composite works that have been prepared through the collaboration of a large number of experts in the various fields represented. Illustrations and tables supplement the material in the essays. Bibliographic references provide information on the sources of the material presented, as well as additional reading for the student in the field.

Specialized works in laboratory analysis abound, and *Methods of Enzymology* represents this type of publication. Each volume (or group of volumes) in the series concentrates on a particular topic, with an editor and a group of contributors providing essays on a state-of-the-art approach. Other ongoing, serial publications carry out the same objectives for their particular specialized areas.

HANDBOOKS RELATED TO CLASSIFICATION AND DIAGNOSIS

9.12 *Manual of the International Statistical Classification of Diseases, Injuries, and Causes of Death.* 2 vols. 9th rev. Geneva, World Health Organization, 1977.

9.13 *The International Classification of Diseases, 9th Revision, Clinical Modification.* 3 vols. Ann Arbor, MI, Edwards, 1978.

9.14 *Diagnostic and Statistical Manual of Mental Disorders.* 3d ed. Washington, DC, American Psychiatric Association, 1980.

9.15 Berkow, Robert, ed. *The Merck Manual of Diagnosis and Therapy.* 13th ed. Rahway, NJ, Merck, 1977.

The *Manual of the International Statistical Classification of Diseases, Injuries, and Causes of Death* represents "a system of categories to which morbid entities are assigned according to some established criteria" (Introduction). These categories make it possible for standardization of the collection of data related to diseases, injuries, and causes of death. To facilitate the study of disease, the scheme has been arranged so that specific disease entity has "a separate title in the classification only when its separation is warranted because the frequency of its occurrence, or its importance as a morbid condition, justifies its isolation as a separate category" (Introduction). This element of grouping represents the difference between a classification for statistical purposes and a nomenclature that must be as detailed as possible to provide for all possible names.

The *Classification* is a decimal classification. The three digits preceding the decimal represent the chosen categories in seventeen broad areas; digits following the decimal represent the specific diseases found in each category.

The clinical modification of the *Classification* (ICD-9-CM) represents an attempt to provide a common classification of diseases and related entities to be "used across the country by all agencies, institutions, and geopolitical jurisdictions" (Foreword). The intent of ICD-9-CM is "to serve as a useful tool in the area of classification of morbidity data for indexing of medical records, medical care review, and ambulatory and other medical care programs, as well as for basic health statistics" (Foreword). The greater precision that is needed in the maintenance of clinical records is provided in the modification.

A complementary publication, *Diagnostic and Statistical Manual of Mental Disorders* (DSM-III), has been prepared by the American Psychiatric Association. Based on the section on mental disorders in the *International Classification*, the DSM-III provides specific diagnostic criteria as guides for making each diagnosis.

The *Merck Manual of Diagnosis and Therapy* contains discussion of factors related to rational diagnostic reasoning and effective therapy, including discussions of symptoms and signs. The twenty-four sections are subdivided by chapters going into considerable detail, and the work attempts to serve as a reference guide for the whole range of medical disorders.

These titles represent but a few of the potential titles that could be included in this chapter. Many are standard titles that should be found in all health sciences libraries; others are examples of the kinds of titles available. Because of the types of information contained in handbooks and manuals, they are likely to be used very heavily in providing ready reference information.

REFERENCE

[1]Grogan, Denis. *Science and Technology: An Introduction to the Literature.* 3d ed., rev. London, Clive Bingley, 1976. p. 68.

CHAPTER 10

Drug Information Sources

JULIE KUENZEL KWAN

Drug information is a broad field including all aspects of the actions of drugs and chemicals on living systems. It includes the traditional fields of pharmacology, the study of the therapeutic uses of drugs; pharmacokinetics, the study of the physiological actions of drugs; pharmacy, the compounding, manufacture, and dispensing of drugs; and toxicology, the study of hazardous effects of chemicals.

Drug information questions are directed to librarians from a number of sources. A physician may want to know if a particular symptom or side effect has previously been associated with the administration of a particular drug. An occupational health specialist may want to know if there is a relationship between a clinical symptom and daily exposure to a chemical in the working environment. A pharmacist may want to know the American equivalent of a drug prescribed in a foreign country. A nurse may want more information about a drug being administered to a patient to assist in monitoring the patient's response to the drug. Members of the public frequently ask questions about drugs they are taking or about additives in the food they eat.

The proliferation of therapeutic drugs is a relatively recent phenomenon. The earliest therapeutic agents were primarily plant and animal substances, and mentioned in early materia medica are such things as garlic, juniper berries, and dragon's blood (of plant origin); these were administered usually as extracts, poultices, or powders. Still in use today are drugs from some of these plant sources—for example, digitalis, obtained from foxglove, and morphine, from the opium poppy. Significant advances in organic chemistry provided for the chemical isolation of these therapeutic agents from the plant and animal sources.

Since World War II, especially, the drug industry has grown tremendously. The combination of advanced techniques in chemical synthesis and a better understanding of the underlying causes of diseases resulted in many more therapeutic agents becoming available. A quick comparison of editions of the *Physician's Desk Reference (PDR)*—a guide to prescription drugs for the physician—from the late 1940s with those published today shows dramatic differences. The early editions list such agents as estrogenic substance in oil, liver injection, and desiccated kidney of hogs, while today's edition lists very specific chemical entities. The size of the *PDR* has also greatly increased; the current edition is more than fifteen times larger than the first, suggesting a substantial increase in the number of drugs available and in the information about them. The increasing use of drugs has even resulted in a new field, iatrogenic disease, meaning "physician-induced disease" and referring primarily to clinical problems resulting from the use of therapeutic drugs.

Information about drugs is complex due to governmental regulation. The Food and Drug Administration (FDA) regulates all drugs in interstate commerce and is responsible for overseeing the labeling of drugs and ensuring that they are both safe and effective. The FDA requires the pharmaceutical company to notify prescribing physicians of contraindications (i.e., when *not* to use a drug), warnings, and adverse effects of drugs. Increasingly they are being asked to provide more information on the drug package label. In recent years the Occupational Safety and Health Administration (OSHA) has become increasingly involved in monitoring the effects of chemicals in industrial settings.

The federal government has established strict regulations regarding the introduction of new drugs and the monitoring of drugs already available. When a pharmaceutical company has a chemical entity that it believes has significant therapeutic value, it is required to file an investigational new drug application (IND) with the FDA and to document the studies that show the therapeutic value and safety of the drug. After substantial testing in animals, the IND testing begins in very small groups of human subjects (phase I studies), either volunteers or exceptionally ill patients for whom other remedies have not worked. If these studies prove promising, clinical trials are expanded to include more human subjects (phase II and III studies). When sufficient data have been collected, the pharmaceutical company submits another application to the FDA, a New Drug Application (NDA) with its data on the safety and effectiveness of the drug.

Approval of the NDA means that the drug is approved for marketing and can be prescribed by licensed practitioners within the prescribing laws of the Comprehensive Drug Act of 1970. Prior to this approval, the drug may be used only by certain physicians who have been approved to handle investigational drugs. Unfortunately, this NDA with its documented evidence never becomes a part of the public domain. It is considered to be proprietary information available only to the company and the FDA. However, researchers often publish their experiences with the drug during clinical trials. This material is retrievable through the journal (and report) literature.

GUIDES TO THE LITERATURE

10.1 Sewell, Winifred. *Guide to Drug Information.* Hamilton, IL. Drug Intelligence Publications, 1976.

10.2 Brunn, Alice L. *How to Find Out in Pharmacy: A Guide to Sources of Pharmaceutical Information.* Oxford, Pergamon, 1969.

10.3 Revill, J. P., ed. *Drug Information Sources: A World-Wide Annotated Survey.* Henley-on-Thames, Eng., Gothard House, 1978.

Among the suggested readings is Mary Jo Reilly's *Drug Information*, which explores the need for and use of drug literature by health care professionals. This work can help the beginning librarian put the drug literature into perspective in providing and planning for literature access in the library. Its main value is in its narrative report of the use of drug literature and its analysis of agencies and organizations devoted to organizing and using it. Winifred Sewell's *Guide to Drug Information* is a very helpful guide that goes into greater depth than this chapter and is oriented towards pharmacy students and other health care students as well as librarians. It is particularly helpful for its analysis of types of questions and for its tabular charts, which compare various drug literature tools. Although it has a British emphasis, Brunn's *How to Find Out in Pharmacy* is useful but dated. *Drug Information Sources* is a recent bibliography and directory with little or no explanation of sources, but it is helpful for international drug coverage. It can serve as a beginning source for collection development, particularly if a library feels a special need for the drug literature from a specific country. It includes professional and trade organizations related to the drug field, along with their addresses; a briefly annotated bibliography of drug publications originating in each country; and international publications.

DRUG NOMENCLATURE

One of the major problems in utilizing the drug literature is recognizing the multiplicity of names for a given chemical compound and understanding how reference sources must be approached depending on the type of name. A thorough understanding of these names is essential (see table 10-1). When a pharmaceutical company is investigating a large number of chemicals for possible therapeutic activity, it frequently assigns alphanumeric designations or code names. Often, a code name is the first designation in the primary literature. The chemical name describes the chemical structure of a drug. There are a number of conventions for these chemical names, but in any case, chemical names are often very lengthy and not readily useful in talking or writing about drugs. Consequently, there is a need for a "common" name to describe a drug, something that is not a tongue twister. "Aspirin" or "tetracycline" are examples of these more easily handled names. Common names are called "generic" or "nonproprietary" names. Names used by a manufacturer to describe specific marketed products are called "proprietary," "trade," or "brand" names. Proprietary names are registered trademarks, as are the color, shape, and markings of each pill or capsule. Two or more manufacturers may market the same generic drug, but each company will have its own proprietary name representing its specific product. These products may differ; while the active ingredients are the same, each manufacturer may use different ingredients in compounding the drug or in holding it together. The composition of a pill, other than amounts of active ingredients, is a proprietary or trade secret, but is often available from the manufacturer in cases where a patient has a reaction to the medication.

Another source of confusion is the multiplicity of generic names. Two companies working with the same drug may call it by different nonproprietary names. In the past this practice has led to such confusion that now "official" nonproprietary names are designated. The United States Adopted Names Commission has the authority to declare a generic name as the officially recognized common name in the United States. If another company wants to market a preparation of that drug, it will use this "official" generic name.

The problem is compounded on an international scale. Other countries also have authorized bodies to establish official names; the World Health Organization's *International Nonproprietary Names* attempts to unify official names in all participating countries, but differences still exist. And, because of the strict laws regulating investigational drugs in this country, new drugs are often available much sooner elsewhere. A patient from France, having been prescribed a French drug, may travel to the United States and need a refill of an American equivalent. A British doctor, taking an American medical licensure exam, finds "meperidine" on the examination questions rather than "pethidine," the name to which British doctors are accustomed. Researchers looking for new cardiac drugs may read about practolol and want to know if there is an American equivalent.

The librarian must understand these types of names to use literature sources effectively. Publications originating from commercial sources are usually arranged by proprietary or trade name. Publications from professional associations are usually arranged by nonproprietary or generic name. Books published in other countries use their own official generic names, which are frequently different from the American form. The librarian, presented with a drug name, may not immediately know what type of name it is. The first step is to determine the type of name and then to go to appropriate reference sources.

SOURCES OF DRUG IDENTIFICATION

10.4 Billups, Norman F. ed. *American Drug Index: 1980*. Philadelphia, PA, Lippincott, 1980.

10.5 Griffiths, Mary C., Dickerman, Marie J., and Miller, Lloyd C. *USAN and the USP Dictionary of Drug Names: A Compilation of the United States Adopted Names (USAN) Selected and Released from June 15, 1961, through June 15, 1979, and Other Names for Drugs, Both Current and Retrospective*. Rockville, MD, United States Pharmacopeial Convention, 1979.

10.6 Windholz, Martha et al., eds. *The Merck Index: An Encyclopedia of Chemicals and Drugs*. 9th ed. Rahway, NJ, Merck and Co., 1976.

10.7 *Unlisted Drugs*. New York, NY, Pharmaceutical Division, Special Libraries Association, Vol. 1– , 1949– .

A number of sources should be readily available for finding brief information about drugs, particularly for identifying proprietary and nonproprietary names. The *American Drug Index (ADI)* includes brief information on a large number of drugs; its comprehensive coverage makes it an ideal source for initial consultation. Both proprietary and nonproprietary names are listed in one alphabet. Proprietary name entries include manufacturer's name, generic or chemical names, composition and strength, pharmaceutical forms available, package size, dosage, and a brief indication of use. Nonproprietary name entries include an indication of whether the name is U.S.P. or N.F. (listed in the U.S. Pharmacopeia or National Formulary, which are described below), USAN (U.S. Adopted Name), or BAN (British Adopted Name). Nonproprietary name entries also list proprietary products, which include the drug and a brief description of use. Proprietary names are given for combination drugs—products that contain more than one therapeutic agent—and the *ADI* lists addresses of distributors and contains other useful appendixes.

Another primary source for brief drug information is the *USAN and the USP Dictionary of Drug Names*. This compilation lists the United States Adopted Names (USANs) selected and released since June 15, 1961. More than 1,600 individual USANs are included, as well as 3,100 proprietary names and more than 2,300 code names. For each USAN the following information is provided: year published as a USAN, a pronunciation guide, molecular formula, chemical name, Chemical Abstracts Service (CAS) registry number, pharmacological or therapeutic activity claim, brand names under which the drug is marketed, manufacturer or distributor, and the structural formula. The *USAN and the USP Dictionary of Drug Names* is particularly useful for its inclusion of earlier drug names, and its pronunciation guide is unique. An excellent introduction details the purpose and history of the USAN Council and procedures by which a USAN is established. Caution is required, however: a listing in the *USAN* does not indicate that the drug is marketed in this country; it only means that an official name has been designated.

A source for brief information about all types of chemicals, including drugs, is the *Merck Index*. When this publication began in 1889, it was only a list of products marketed by the Merck Company. Now in its ninth edition, the *Merck Index* has evolved into a comprehensive encyclopedia of chemicals, drugs, and biological substances. The *Merck Index* must be accessed through its index, since cross-references do not exist in the body of the work. In addition to standard information such as chemical name, structural formula, and brief description of use, the *Merck Index* includes references to patents and journal articles describing the preparation of the chemical. An index of chemical names gives the corresponding CAS registry numbers. Rounding out this work's utility as a general reference source, there are several appendixes, including organic named reactions, tables of radioactive isotopes, and mathematical tables.

A unique tool in the drug literature is a serial publication called *Unlisted Drugs*. Begun in 1949 by the Pharmaceutical Division of the Special Libraries Association, this publication was designed to bridge the gap between standard reference texts and reports of new drugs in the periodical literature. Drugs are considered "unlisted" when they are not included in several major works such as the *American Drug Index* or the *Merck Index*, referred to by the producers of *Unlisted Drugs* as "exclusion sources." Currently the exclusion sources for *Unlisted Drugs* are the latest editions of the *American Drug Index* and the *Merck Index* (already described), *Martindale's Extra Pharmacopoeia* (to be described), the *Rote Liste* (a listing of drug products marketed in Germany), the *Vidal Dictionnaire* (French-marketed products), and *Unlisted Drugs* back to its first issue.

Unlisted Drugs gives only brief information on each drug, including composition, manufacturer, pharmacological action, and a literature citation. Sometimes the structural formula is given. Earlier references to listings in *Unlisted Drugs* are also included, as well as any equivalent forms when available. *Unlisted Drugs* is also available in card format.

Another feature of *Unlisted Drugs* is its excellent book review section. New books from around the world are listed and summarized; coverage is particularly useful to the pharmaceutical industry, since even very expensive marketing research reports are included. As an adjunct service, *Unlisted Drugs* offers a book ordering service so that smaller libraries do not have to deal directly with individual publishers to obtain the materials. A core collection in drug nomenclature might include *Unlisted Drugs* and its exclusion sources. A cumulated index, the *Unlisted Drugs Index Guide*, cumulates all entries since the first volume; now in its fourth edition covering 1947 to 1976, it contains over 90,000 entries, making it an excellent source for old and new drugs.

COMPREHENSIVE TREATISES AND TEXTBOOKS

10.8   Goodman, Louis S., and Gilman, Alfred. *The Pharmacological Basis of Therapeutics*. 5th ed. New York, NY, Macmillan, 1975.

10.9   Wade, Ainley, ed. *Martindale: The Extra Pharmacopoeia*. 27th ed. London, Pharmaceutical Press, 1977.

10.10 Osol, Arthur, et al., eds. *Remington's Pharmaceutical Sciences: A Treatise on the Theory and Practice of Pharmaceutical Sciences, with Essential Information about Pharmaceutical and Medicinal Agents.* 15th ed. Easton, PA, Mack, 1975.

The previously mentioned sources do not give extensive information about drugs, but they do identify whether a drug name is proprietary or nonproprietary and give some indication of the manufacturer of a drug. Armed with this brief information, the librarian may wish to consult next a more comprehensive source, which usually will give a detailed description of the drug's pharmacological action.

Goodman and Gilman's *The Pharmacological Basis of Therapeutics* has long been considered the "blue Bible of pharmacology." It has been a standard text in medical and pharmacy schools, although there is some opinion now that due to its vast encyclopedic nature it serves best as a reference tool, while students need texts outlining the philosophical and practical principles of drug therapy. Still, it remains an extremely valuable treatise of drug information. The first chapter is concerned with general principles, after which chapters are arranged by mode of action—for example, drugs acting on the central nervous system, anesthetics, and cardiovascular drugs. Drugs with a long history of use, such as curare, morphine, and penicillin, have brief histories. The bulk of the material, however, relates to pharmacologic action, with emphasis placed on comparisons of similarly acting drugs.

Martindale's Extra Pharmacopoeia provides similar in-depth information and is also arranged by drug classes. Each drug monograph is lengthy, including pharmacological action and adverse effects. Because regulations regarding new drugs are not as stringent in other countries as they are in the United States, Martindale's international coverage includes many drugs not available here. Since this is a British publication, the monographs are listed under British Adopted Names, but other official names, including USANs, are given immediately thereafter when available. Following each monograph is an indication of proprietary forms, identifying the marketed names and countries of origin. An extensive index correlates all nonproprietary and proprietary names.

The third source, Remington's *Pharmaceutical Sciences,* provides extensive information from a pharmaceutical viewpoint. Used as a text in many pharmacy schools, Remington's includes information on specific drugs as well as information on the practice of pharmacy and pharmacy laws (for example, the Comprehensive Drug Act of 1970).

COMMERCIAL SOURCES OF DRUG INFORMATION

10.11 *Physicians' Desk Reference*. 34th ed. Oradell, NJ, Medical Economics, 1980.

10.12 *PharmIndex: Professional Product Information for Pharmacists*. Portland, OR, Skyline Publishers. 1958– . Looseleaf.

There are a number of sources that give information about specific marketed products. The pharmaceutical manufacturer is responsible for providing certain basic information, the content of which is approved by the Food and Drug Administration. One mechanism by which the manufacturer informs the physician about a specific product is the "package insert," a brief brochure that generally includes the proprietary and chemical names; pharmacological action; indications and contraindications; warnings, precautions, and adverse reactions; dosage and overdosage; dosage forms; and, in most cases, references. The package insert is not necessarily complete or balanced. Although the FDA has agreed to the manufacturer's statements about the product, the package insert remains a publicity and promotion mechanism for the manufacturer. Although the manufacturer is legally responsible for the correctness of information included, a package insert does not compare or evaluate a given drug with other agents.

Information from package inserts is published annually in the *PDR: Physicians' Desk Reference*. Information in the *PDR* is arranged by company name with many, but not all, marketed products listed. It is particularly useful for dosage, composition of each product, contraindications, warnings, use, and adverse effects. Indexes are by brand name, type of action or preparation, and generic, chemical, and manufacturer's name. Also included is a picture section of the most frequently marketed products. The physical representation of capsules and tablets is registered for each manufacturer just as the names are trademarked. This is a useful source for identifying pills and capsules in unlabeled containers. Since the *PDR* is a source of manufacturer disclaimer, side effects are enumerated in great detail, but often no indication is given of the severity or frequency of the side effects. Since the manufacturing industry cannot conduct safety tests in pregnant humans, for example, the work is liberally peppered with the statement, "Safety of this drug during pregnancy is unknown."

The earliest editions of the *PDR* carried the subtitle "for the physician's desk only." But with the recent consumer movement in health care, this statement has been removed, and the *PDR* is now for sale throughout the country in bookstore chains serving the general public. Many health care consumers regularly ask health science librarians for the *PDR,* and the public's reliance on this tool should be a topic of general concern to librarians. First, the information is not necessarily unbiased but represents only what the FDA has approved the manufacturer to say. Second, the information is technical and difficult for the layman to understand. Perhaps one of the greatest challenges to the health sciences librarian is to channel members of the public from the *PDR* to more appropriate sources for their use.

PharmIndex is a monthly looseleaf publication specifically designed for the pharmacist. It is arranged by proprietary name and lists virtually every product on the market. The information is brief and includes packaging and price information. *PharmIndex* presents a section on investigational drugs in its products pending section (which includes published references), as well as information on new or changed products.

PROFESSIONAL SOURCES OF DRUG INFORMATION

10.13 *American Hospital Formulary Service.* Washington, DC, American Society of Hospital Pharmacists. 1959– . 2 vols. Looseleaf.

10.14 AMA Department of Drugs. *AMA Drug Evaluations.* 4th ed. Littleton, MA, Publishing Sciences Group, 1979.

10.15 *Accepted Dental Therapeutics.* 38th ed. Chicago, IL, Council on Dental Therapeutics, American Dental Association, 1980.

10.16 *Handbook of Nonprescription Drugs.* 6th ed. Washington, DC, American Pharmaceutical Association, 1979.

Some of the best sources of drug information originate from professional societies. Their chief benefit lies in their authoritative evaluation. Professional groups such as the American Society for Hospital Pharmacists and the American Medical Association compile and evaluate information for their members. These tools are extremely valuable in the library setting.

The *American Hospital Formulary Service* is a two-volume looseleaf service produced by the American Society of Hospital Pharmacists. It is designed to be a current collection of unbiased and evaluated monographs (hence the looseleaf format) for pharmacists and other members of the medical community. The *Formulary Service* is arranged by class of drug, for example, antineoplastic agents, cardiovascular drugs, hormones, and synthetic substitutes. Each section, tabbed for convenience in use, begins with a listing of the generic names found in that section. This listing can be helpful when spellings are doubtful. For example, a medical student interested in "decarbazine," an antineoplastic agent, in consulting the *Formulary Service,* would find the correct spelling, "dacarbazine." Each monograph includes alternate names; chemical structural formula; descriptive sections on pharmacology, absorption, distribution, metabolism, and excretion; uses; cautions; dosage; and proprietary preparations including this agent. Although the looseleaf format allows easy updating, this format is also the book's biggest drawback. Pages can be easily removed (pages on opiate drugs tend to disappear swiftly), and some type of protective mechanism should be used to keep the pages intact, either by keeping an archival copy off the general shelves or collating pages after each use.

Investigational uses of approved drugs are included, as are some nonprescription agents such as vitamins. Many sections have an introductory statement about the class of drugs; for example, the section on radiopharmaceuticals has a general statement about the physics of radioactivity, radiation effects, and radiation protection. A classification number is assigned to each drug, and in the index both nonproprietary and proprietary names refer to classification number. Supplements are issued several times a year.

AMA Drug Evaluations is a joint effort of the American Medical Association Department of Drugs and the American Society for Clinical Pharmacology and Therapeutics. It is intended to correlate current scientific findings on drugs and relate them to the wisdom of experienced clinicians. *AMA Drug Evaluations* gives uses, routes of administration, and dosages, which may or may not be found in the package insert. The labeling laws of the FDA limit the marketing and advertising of drugs but do not limit the use of the drug for an individual patient at the physician's discretion. Therefore, *AMA Drug Evaluations* attempts to describe all scientifically recognized uses of a given agent regardless of the package insert. Again, information in this work is arranged by therapeutic class. Each section begins with general statements on the conditions requiring treatment and then gives individual evaluations of various drugs used in treatment, including dosage and preparations available. Two notable aspects are the evaluation of mixtures of drugs and the emphasis on the treatment of a condition or disease, including related material on diet. A supplementary chapter deals with drugs affecting the results of common laboratory tests. There are two indexes, an adverse reaction index and a drugs index.

Accepted Dental Therapeutics is a comparable publication published by the American Dental Association to assist dentists in using drugs in practice, to alert them to new drugs that may be potentially useful in dentistry, and to inform them of problems arising in dental treatment in patients who may be taking medications for other medical problems. Information is arranged by therapeutic use, such as agents for anxiety control, local anesthetics, and antimicrobial agents.

The *Handbook of Nonprescription Drugs,* published by the American Pharmaceutical Association, deals only with over-the-counter (OTC) or nonprescription products. Although the lay public assumes that no harm can come from the use of nonprescription drugs, in reality there are certain dangers, and this book addresses that fact. Each chapter deals with a therapeutic use—for example, laxative products, infant formula products, contact lens products, sunscreen products—in short, any products which may be purchased without prescription. The chapters describe the condition and the mechanism of action of available products. Often they include charts comparing the preparations. Before OTC product manufacturers were required to list all ingredients on the label, this source was useful for comparative purposes, for example, to determine which shampoos contain hexachlorophene. While it is still useful for this purpose, it is perhaps most utilized now for its overview of nonprescription remedies.

OFFICIAL COMPENDIA

10.17 *The United States Pharmacopeia.* Twentieth Revision. *The National Formulary.* Fifteenth Edition. Rockville, MD, United States Pharmacopeial Convention, Inc., 1979.

10.18 *United States Pharmacopeia Dispensing Information.* Rockville, MD, United States Pharmacopeial Convention, Inc., 1980.

A pharmacopeia is an official book of legal pharmaceutical standards. Countries publish pharmacopeias to define the purity and standards of chemicals used in therapy. Often included are references to chemical tests and assay methods. The two official compendia recognized in the United States are the *U. S. Pharmacopeia (USP)* and the *National Formulary (NF).* These two publications have both been publishing official standards since 1820 and 1888, respectively, although under different sponsorship. After publication of the *National Formulary XIV,* the *NF* was acquired by the U.S. Pharmacopeial Convention, and in 1979, the twentieth revision of the *United States Phar-macopeia* and the fifteenth edition of the *National Formulary* were published in one volume. A new publication, the *United States Phar-macopeia Dispensing Information,* was introduced to provide prescrib-ing and dispensing information not included in the official compen-dia, for example, precautions, side effects, and dosage. Two drug monograph sections are included, one written for the health care provider and one written in lay language to be used as an aid to patient consultation.

The *U. S. Pharmacopeia* and *National Formulary* contain much useful information, but pharmacopeias from other countries are actually little needed by most health sciences librarians in the United States unless users in a particular library require a heavy emphasis on phar-macy and the manufacture of drugs. The need to collect pharmaco-peias from other countries is, in fact, often misinterpreted. Most drug questions relate to therapeutic use or to the general identification of a drug, rather than to standards of purity as given in these compendia. However, caution should be exercised in evaluating any title includ-ing the word "pharmacopeia." *Martindale's Extra Pharmacopoeia,* for example, is not really a pharmacopeia in the true sense of the word, since it is not a listing of legal standards. For those libraries with a demonstrated need for pharmacopeias, *Drug Information Sources* is a handy selection tool.

ADVERSE EFFECTS, TOXICOLOGY, POISONING, AND DRUG ABUSE

10.19 *Meyler's Side Effects of Drugs: A Survey of Unwanted Effects of Drugs.* Amsterdam, Excerpta Medica, 1952–75. 8 vols.

10.20 *Side Effects of Drugs Annual: a Worldwide Yearly Survey of New Data and Trends.* Amsterdam, Excerpta Medica. Vol. 1– . 1977– .

10.21 *Registry of Toxic Effects of Chemical Substances.* Cincinnati, OH, National Institute for Occupational Safety and Health, 1977. Microfiche.

10.22 Gosselin, Robert E., et al. *Clinical Toxicology of Commercial Products: Acute Poisoning.* 4th ed. Baltimore, MD, Williams & Wilkins, 1976.

10.23 Sax, N. Irving. *Dangerous Properties of Industrial Materials.* 5th ed. New York, NY, Van Nostrand, Reinhold, 1979.

Some of the most commonly asked questions concern the untoward effects of drugs and chemicals. "What are the adverse effects of indomethacin?" "What is the lethal dose of aspirin?" "My child drank a bottle of laundry starch—what should I do?" A number of previously described sources give some of this information, but other tools should also be considered.

Side Effects of Drugs includes comprehensive review articles that summarize side effects of drugs reported in the international literature. The information is selective and reviewed critically, and indexes provide access from proprietary names, nonproprietary names, and type of side effect. After publication of the eighth volume, *Side Effects of Drugs Annual* was introduced to provide more timely publication.

The Registry of Toxic Effects of Chemical Substances (RTECS) is prepared by the National Institute for Occupational Safety and Health (NIOSH) to identify all known toxic substances in our environment and to codify known toxic doses. It is arranged by chemical substance, and the following information is included when available: CAS registry number, molecular weight and formula, toxic dose data, and United States and NIOSH documents citing standards for handling these substances. The toxic dose data include dose, route of administration or exposure, kind of effect, and published reference. Approximately 21,000 chemicals are listed.

Clinical Toxicology of Commercial Products is specifically designed to give toxicity and hazard information for chemicals contained in products used in the home and in the commercial setting. For example, it gives information on oven cleaners, hair spray, and the artificial snow used to spray Christmas trees. A wide variety of products is included, with special sections on ingredients, trade names, and representative formulas. In addition, a special section on first aid and emergency care is provided, as are descriptions of therapeutic measures for selected classes of ingredients.

Dangerous Properties of Industrial Materials rates various industrial chemicals giving the chemical name, synonyms, molecular formula, and hazard analysis (toxicity, radiation hazards, and fire hazards). For example, vinyl chloride, a chemical frequently used in processing industries, is listed with a high hazard rating for exposure through inhalation. Countermeasures are listed: adequate ventilation in working with vinyl chloride is necessary. Also included are recommendations for storage and handling and for shipping.

This discussion would not be complete without a brief mention of poison control centers. The first poison control center was opened in 1953; since then additional centers have been established. The National Clearinghouse for Poison Control Centers collects information on poisons and disseminates this information throughout the country. The services of these centers are available to all physicians, and their aim is to provide prompt information on poisoning and its treatment. Standard reference works such as the *PDR* often include listings of poison control centers.

DRUG INTERACTIONS

10.24 *Evaluations of Drug Interactions.* 2d ed. Washington, DC, American Pharmaceutical Association, 1976.

10.25 Hansten, Philip D. *Drug Interactions: Clinical Significance of Drug-Drug Interactions and Drug Effects on Clinical Laboratory Results.* 4th ed. Philadelphia, PA, Lea & Febiger, 1979.

A new and increasingly important area of drug information concerns the literature of drug interactions. It is becoming more evident that administering a drug coincidentally with another drug or chemical can affect the pharmacological action. For example, procarbazine should not be taken with cheese or wine. Some drugs can potentiate or speed up the action of another drug. Some drugs may effectively lose any therapeutic potential if taken with another drug. Clearly, these interrelationships must be better understood and codified.

ABSTRACTING AND INDEXING SERVICES AND ONLINE DATA BASES

10.26 *Drug Literature Index.* Amsterdam, Excerpta Medica. Vol. 1– , 1969– .

10.27 *International Pharmaceutical Abstracts: Key to the World's Literature of Pharmacy.* Washington, DC, American Society of Hospital Pharmacists. Vol. 1– , 1964– .

10.28 *Inpharma: Weekly Reports form the Current International Drug Literature.* Balgowlah, Australia, ADIS Press. No. 1– , 1975– .

Although abstracting and indexing services and online data bases are described elsewhere, a few comments should be made regarding drug information questions, and some abstracting and indexing services specific to drug information should be noted.

The National Library of Medicine's *Medical Subject Headings (MeSH)* has shown a dramatic increase in its inclusion of drug names since its inception. Earliest editions relied heavily on classes of chemical compounds. Each year, however, many specific drug names have been added to Section D, "Chemicals and Drugs." In fact, approximately half of the new *MeSH* headings added every year are drugs and chemicals, so that the 1980 edition of *MeSH* includes more than 5,500 headings for chemicals and drugs.

All *MeSH* entries for drugs are nonproprietary names. In a few cases, when the proprietary name is very common, there is a cross-reference from the proprietary name to the nonproprietary *MeSH* heading. Therefore, for the user of *Index Medicus*, tools such as the *American Drug Index* or the *USAN and the USP Dictionary of Drug Names* may often be needed to convert a proprietary name to a nonproprietary name. Sometimes, the drug name may be a minor descriptor, and it will be necessary to use a broader name, representing a class of drugs, to find information in the printed *Index Medicus*. The user must pay special attention to entry dates for *MeSH* headings, since drug names have been added so frequently to *MeSH*.

Often is it useful to determine when a drug became an official USAN. This will give an indication of a realistic time period for a search. For example, ribavirin, a relatively new antiviral agent, became a USAN in 1974 and a provisional *MeSH* heading in 1975. To search *Index Medicus*, one would look under the heading "ribonucleosides," since the term *ribavirin* is only a provisional heading. Since other ribonucleosides are indexed in the same place, one would next scan for article titles that mention ribavirin or its proprietary name, Virazole. For a MEDLINE search, "ribavirin" will suffice back through 1975, but for previous years, especially before 1974 when the USAN was approved, the search would have to include the proprietary name.

In other cases, information may be needed about the drug therapy of a specific disease or chemicals causing a disease. In these cases, the subheadings "drug therapy" and "chemically induced" are especially useful in searching both *Index Medicus* and MEDLINE. The librarian should be familiar with all the subheadings applicable to Section D of *MeSH*.

The Excerpta Medica abstracting services have two specific drug-related sections, *Pharmacology and Toxicology* and *Drug Dependence*. Other sections, for example, *Cancer* and *Internal Medicine*, include numerous articles on therapeutic agents used in these specialties. The Excerpta Medica Foundation has repackaged all drug-related articles in the *Drug Literature Index*, which has special indexes for classification codes, pharmaceutical or nonproprietary names, proprietary or trade names, new drugs, and author names. In a parallel manner, the on-line version of *Excerpta Medica*, which includes the *Drug Literature Index*, can be searched through the proprietary name field.

Chemical Abstracts, another source described earlier, is also a useful source of information. Many of the biochemistry sections include drug information material. See, for example, sections on pharmaco-dynamics, hormone pharmacology, toxicology, and biochemical interactions. In the macromolecular chemistry sections there are two of interest, pharmaceuticals and pharmaceutical analysis. Many of the sections relating to industrial chemistry include references to occupational hazards. When searching *Chemical Abstracts* for a particular drug, the *Index Guide* should be consulted to find the correct index term. Specific chemicals are included in the *Chemical Substance Index*. Ribavirin, for example, is indexed under 1H-1, 2,4-triazole-3-carbox-amide, $- 1-\beta$-D-ribofuranosyl$-$. Classes of chemicals or other concepts, such as "antibiotics" and "brain neoplasms," are indexed in the *General Subject Index*. Because of its great breadth, *Chemical Abstracts* is often used to locate citations not findable elsewhere. Patents describing the manufacture of a specific drug fall in this category. While the emphasis is not primarily on clinical medicine, extensive research material is included.

The semimonthly *International Pharmaceutical Abstracts (IPA)* covers many areas of interest to pharmacists and drug information specialists, including pharmaceutical technology, the practice of pharmacy, investigational drugs, drug testing and analysis, drug stability, and pharmaceutical chemistry. The journal coverage includes many basic medical journals, and many sources not included in *Index Medicus*. Examples of the latter include *Drug Intelligence and Clinical Pharmacy*, *American Druggist*, the *Federal Register*, and the *FDA Drug Bulletin*. The *IPA* is useful for finding information on topics such as drug sales, drug information services, and chemical information such as the half-life or stability of a drug.

A relatively new publication, *Inpharma: Weekly Reports from the Current International Drug Literature*, has been published since 1975 by ADIS Press. This publication provides descriptive abstracts of very recent articles on drugs in clinical use; its chief value is as a current alerting tool for pharmacists and others involved in drug therapy. Most issues include a section on drugs newly introduced in various countries of the world and summary listings of articles on selected topics. Librarians will find this an excellent source to recommend and use, since it provides more current information than *Index Medicus.* There are monthly, six-month, and annual indexes to *Inpharma* by nonproprietary name, disease state, and general terms such as hepatotoxicity and pregnancy. New product introductions are cumulated, and drug interactions are combined under one heading.

TOXLINE, described elsewhere as a prime tool to locate toxicology information, also includes a variety of nontoxicologic information. Its inclusion of the pharmacodynamics section of *Chemical Abstracts* and the *International Pharmaceutical Abstracts* makes it an ideal source of general drug information. Searching *Chemical Abstracts* online will retrieve materials not included in the sections of *Chemical Abstracts* included in TOXLINE. The librarian must keep in mind that a key source in deciding to search TOXLINE versus *Chemical Abstracts,* is the *Subject Coverage and Arrangement of Abstracts by Section in Chemical Abstracts,* which outlines Chemical Abstracts Service's scope policies.

Other NLM data bases of interest to drug specialists include CHEMLINE, RTECS, CANCERLIT, and CLINPROT. CHEMLINE can be used quite effectively when constructing search terms for natural language data bases, including TOXLINE. The on-line version of *RTECS* (*Registry of Toxic Effects of Chemical Substances*) is much easier to use than the printed version, and it is more timely. CANCERLIT, developed by the International Cancer Research Data Bank (ICRDB) of the National Cancer Institute, is the online version of *Carcinogenesis Abstracts* and *Cancer Therapy Abstracts.* Since it is a natural language data base, it is most useful for searches involving words in titles or abstracts and for searches relating to cancer alone. For example, MOPP is an acronym for the four-drug combination of nitrogen mustard (*m*echlorethamine), vincristine (*O*ncovin), *p*rocarbazine, and *p*rednisone. Note that this combination acronym includes initials for both proprietary and nonproprietary names. Another data base developed by the ICRDB, CLINPROT (*Clin*ical *Prot*ocols), is a register of clinical investigations of new anticancer agents and treatment methods. Since the drugs included are investigational, they may not be fully reported elsewhere.

FOREIGN DRUGS

10.29 Marler, E. E. J. *Pharmacological and Chemical Synonyms: A Collection of Drugs, Pesticides, and Other Compounds Drawn from the Literature of the World.* 6th ed. Amsterdam, Excerpta Medica, 1976.

10.30 *Index Nominum: 1980.* 10th ed. Zurich, Société Suisse de Pharmacie, 1979.

Foreign drug questions are a particularly vexing problem because, no matter how extensive a particular drug reference collection is, there always seem to be drugs about which the librarians simply cannot locate information. In addition, spelling may vary in different languages. Many times users have insufficient information, and the librarian begins a search looking for the proverbial needle in the haystack. Whenever possible, the requester should be queried for further information by means of questions such as: Do you have the exact spelling of the drug name? Do you know the country of origin? What is the drug used for?

Several sources described earlier are very useful for foreign drug names. The *Merck Index,* because of its broad international coverage and its inclusion of many proprietary and nonproprietary names, is an excellent first source. *Martindale's Extra Pharmacopoeia* is also extremely valuable for its extensive coverage of European drugs. *Unlisted Drugs,* because of its broad coverage and the ease of covering many years through the *Unlisted Drug Index Guide,* should also be consulted.

Two other sources that are useful for foreign drug identification are Marler's *Pharmacological and Chemical Synonyms* and *Index Nominum.* Marler attempts to include all drug names but does not give any information other than corresponding proprietary and nonproprietary names. *Index Nominum,* which is published in French, goes a bit further. All listings are under the World Health Organization's international nonproprietary name with the following information: chemical name, structural formula, therapeutic class, generic names, official names, and proprietary names. Unfortunately, this listing is not complete, and in some cases the USANs have been omitted, diminishing its utility in American libraries.

Online services often can be used advantageously for foreign drug names. These names may appear in the title or in the abstract, and with the case of the Excerpta Medica system, there is a field specifically designated for proprietary names. With the online systems, it is possible to "neighbor" a term to see if there are variant spellings. Author addresses and use of the drug may also help in identification.

DRUG INFORMATION FOR PATIENTS AND THE PUBLIC

As indicated previously, the consumer movement in the United States has greatly increased the public's "desire to know." Health sciences librarians are frequently asked drug information questions by the general public, and accordingly each library must decide its own policy for responding to these questions. Most materials are very technical, and the general writing style usually does not lend itself to easy interpretation. The librarian should always exercise discretion and encourage requesters to consult with a physician or pharmacist to interpret and evaluate their questions.

No matter how thoroughly a physician or nurse describes a medication to a patient, errors in use do occur. One study[1] indicated that over 80% of the patients incorrectly administered their medications. More and more frequently, instructions and warnings are included in drug packaging, most notably with oral contraceptives.

Patient package inserts might prove to be an effective method of health education for the patient, reinforcing the physician's verbal directions. These inserts could tell the patient what the drug is, what it is used for, what side effects to watch for, and when to contact the physician. Obviously, the content and readability of such inserts would be critical. Consider, for example, the following directions for Valium at the eleventh-grade readability level versus the fifth-grade readability level.

Eleventh-grade level
Coadministration of this medication with alcoholic beverages or other CNS depressing drugs (e.g., sedatives, tranquilizers, antihistamines, etc.) may add to the sedative effect.

Fifth-grade level
You should not take this drug while you are drinking alcoholic beverages, such as wine or beer. You should avoid taking this drug with other medications you may be taking for sleep or tension.[2]

Although patient package inserts are being hotly debated at the present time, what a boon it would be for the health sciences librarian to have a "Patient's Desk Reference" to offer when a member of the public asks for the *PDR!*

DRUG INFORMATION SERVICES

As pharmacists' roles are expanding from the mere dispensing of medications to more active participation in patient care, more hospitals are forming special drug information services that provide specialized information about drugs to the medical and nursing staffs. Pharmacists working in the drug information service will answer detailed questions arising during patient care, will provide a continuing educational medium by reviewing publications on drugs, and often will extend their services to other health professionals in the community.

These drug information services often utilize reference sources that only very specialized libraries might carry. One such specialized tool is a series of card services formerly produced by Paul de Haen, Inc., now produced by MicroMedix, Inc., providing detailed information about drugs being marketed and investigational drugs. Another specialized service is the Iowa Drug Information Service, which utilizes microfiche and a computer index that includes copies of texts of original articles.

If a drug information service is located in a hospital or community, the librarian should find out what it provides. Librarians should be able to show library users how to find drug-related information and refer to the drug information service evaluative or interpretive questions.

REFERENCES

[1]Leary, J. A., Vessela, D. M., and Yeaw, E. M. Self-administered medications. *Amer. J. Nurs.* 71:1193–1194, June 1971.

[2]Bast, L. Peter and Angaran, David M. Johnny can't read. *Drug Intell. Clin. Pharm.* 12:485, August 1978.

READINGS

Anzlowar, Boris R., and Sewell, Winifred. Unlisted Drugs: Evolution of a Cooperative Drug Information Service. *Proc. Drug Inf. Assoc.* 2:59–68, 1966.

Closson, Richard. Foreign Drug Identification. *Drug Intell. Clin. Pharm.* 8: 437–443, July 1974.

Cohen, Marsha N. What Drug Information Should the Consumer Have? Consumer Perspective. *Drug Inf. J.* 11:34–38, Jan/Mar 1977.

Ellis, Joan. Useful Sources of Foreign Drug Information. *Drug Inf. J.* 9:110–113, May/Sep 1975.

Groth, Paul E. Government and Drug Information—the FDA. *Drug Inf. J.* 12:33–36, Jan/Mar 1978.

Reilly, Mary Jo. *Drug Information: Literature Review of Needs, Resources, and Services.* Rockville, MD, Health Services and Mental Health Administration, 1972. (*DHEW* Publication No. (H SM) 72-3031).

Urdang, George. The Development of Pharmacopeias: A Review with Special Reference to the *Pharmacopoeia Internationalis. Bull. WHO* 4:577–603, 1951.

Weindling, Nelson. Statistical Sources for Pharmacists. *J. Am. Pharm. Assoc.* 14:26–30, 40, Jan 1974.

Table 1 Types of drug names

Research code names: Ro 5-0690
                        NSC-115748

Chemical name: 3H-1, 4-Benzodiazepin-2-amine, 7-chloro-N-methyl-

                  5-phenyl, 4-oxide, monohydrochloride

Nonproprietary name: Chlordiazepoxide hydrochloride

Official name: Chlordiazepoxide hydrochloride

Proprietary names: Librium (Hoffman-LaRoche)
                      SK-Lygen (Smith, Kline and French)

CAS registry number: 438-41-5

Structural formula:

CHAPTER 11

Audiovisual Reference Sources

J. MICHAEL HOMAN

CHARACTERISTICS OF AUDIOVISUAL COLLECTIONS IN HEALTH SCIENCES LIBRARIES

Audiovisual collections in health sciences libraries and learning resource centers can be characterized in general as "working collections"
that are curriculum based and, as such, are used to support or supplement educational programs within the institution. Most health
science media collections never become "archival collections," since
very few institutions can justify the expense associated with the
acquisition or local production of audiovisual materials (AVs) not
related to an ongoing educational program. Although AVs continue
to be used extensively to document biomedical research, only the
very largest media collections ever become archival research collections capable, for instance, of supporting research into techniques of
heart surgery recorded on film over the past twenty-five years. In a
working collection there is heavy reliance on recent material, due to
continuous changes in curricula resulting from new knowledge or
through changes in educational goals or institutional priorities. As a
rule, AVs added to working collections have been evaluated prior to
purchase; because the approach to and the methods used for teaching
a particular topic often differ markedly from one institution to another.

CHARACTERISTICS OF AUDIOVISUAL REFERENCE WORK

Audiovisuals are produced in different formats, with different running times, aimed at different audience levels, and obtained from a variety of sources. These and other characteristics are important considerations when one is attempting to satisfy an audiovisual reference request. Categorization of these items on an AV reference request form may be beneficial. In many situations, this categorization will jog the librarian's memory as to what points should be clarified before proceeding with the request.

A general AV request form appears in figure 11-1. Important characteristics that appear on the request form include: intended audience, media format, equipment specifications, procurement method, running time, physical requirements such as color and sound, and cost limits for purchase or rental. Overlooking any of these characteristics will undoubtedly result in an unsatisfied patron. For example, since health science AVs are generally produced with a specific purpose in mind—e.g., professional continuing education, in-service training, patient education—the intended audience should be identified before a reference search is conducted. Nothing is more frustrating to the patron and the librarian than to locate a media program on the correct topic only to discover later that the audience was misidentified. Identification of particular format is also important because some formats (e.g., filmstrips) have limited applications or employ unconventional playback equipment.

A variety of formats may be encountered during a reference search, partly because the format complements the content and purpose of the program. The audiocassette format, for example, has been popular for many years for current awareness (e.g., cassettes produced by Audio Digest), while the videocassette format is used extensively for professional continuing education (e.g., programs produced by Network for Continuing Medical Education). Slide sets with accompanying audiocassettes are popular with undergraduate groups or for self-study. If motion is required, the motion picture format (16mm, 8mm, Super 8mm) or the videotape format (¾-inch U-matic) is often used.

The format is important not only for content and purpose, but also for the situation in which the program will be used. A filmstrip, for example, may be an appropriate format for an individual or small group, but for a large group it would be totally inappropriate. Excel-

Figure 11-1. Sample AV reference request form

AV INFORMATION REQUEST

Date _____
Date required _____

NAME _____ ADDRESS _____
_____

PHONE NUMBER _____
STATUS _____ DEPARTMENT _____ ACC'T. NO. _____
_____

Please indicate the nature of the information that you need. Be as specific as possible. Define any terms that may have special meanings. If applicable list any areas or points not to be included in the search. (Use the back for more space.)

If applicable circle any of the following areas of primary interest:

Etiology   Pathology   Diagnosis   Treatment   Technique   Prevention   Other _____

USE DATE _____ HOW LONG NEEDED _____ INTENDED AUDIENCE _____
_____ USED BY GROUPS _____ INDIVIDUALS _____
MATERIAL WILL BE RENTED _____ , PURCHASED _____ .
HOW MUCH WILL YOU PAY FOR: RENTAL _____ PURCHASE _____ PREVIEW _____
_____ CHECK IF ONLY FREE MATERIALS CAN BE ACCEPTED.

SEARCH RESTRICTIONS:

	FORMAT:	____ 16 mm films	____ 8mm films	____ Filmstrips
		____ Slides	____ Video-recording	____ Transparencies
	LENGTH:	____ Less than 15 minutes	____ 30 to 45 minutes	
		____ 15 to 30 minutes	____ More than 45 minutes	

lent discussions of the various media formats and the pros and cons of each may be found in a number of the suggested readings following this chapter.

The procurement method and physical characteristics of a program are also important factors in a reference search. A number of procurement methods exist for health science AVs. These include purchase, free loan, rent, interlibrary loan, and duplication. The procurement method chosen will depend on the intended use of the item. A program to be used once as an adjunct to a lecture should be borrowed or rented rather than purchased. Likewise, the identification of a fifty-minute 16mm movie would not be appropriate were it requested in conjunction with a forty-five minute lecture.

BIBLIOGRAPHIC CONTROL OF NONPRINT MATERIALS

The successful location of relevant software is severely hindered by the lack of bibliographic control that characterizes AV production in the health sciences. There is no national bibliography equivalent to *Books in Print* for audiovisual material in the health sciences, and there is as yet no bibliography of bibliographies for available reference tools. Libraries desiring comprehensive coverage of AV productions are currently forced to collect hundreds of producer and distributor catalogs from commercial, educational, and governmental institutions. It is estimated that there are currently more than 600 producers and distributors of health science media. To compound the problem, the individual catalogs or brochures that must be collected differ substantially as to the quality and quantity of bibliographic information they contain. In a survey of distributor catalogs, McIlvaine and Brantz[1] found that only 40–60% of the distributor catalogs in their sample contained information about the intended audience, date of production, or producer, and that 25% or fewer provided a title or subject index.

A number of reference tools have been published to help alleviate the bibliographic control problem, but none of them, including the publications resulting from the National Library of Medicine (NLM)'s AVLINE data base, provides comprehensive coverage at the present time. There is good reason to be sanguine about the future of bibliographic control, however, judging from recent efforts to persuade media producers to make available in a standardized format those elements necessary for effective bibliographic control of media.

Spencer and Schiffer,[2] working through the Biomedical Libraries Section of the Health Sciences Communications Association (HeSCA), published a list of descriptive cataloging elements for use in the bibliographic control of nonprint materials in the *Journal of Biocommunication*, an important AV production-oriented journal published by HeSCA and the Association of Medical Illustrators. The authors based their list of cataloging elements on the *Anglo-American Cataloging Rules*, chapter 12, revised *(AACR)*.[3] The list of descriptive cataloging elements was meant to serve as a guideline for standardized bibliographic descriptions of nonprint publications; *AACR II* expands upon these basic principles. Bogen,[4] in an article also appearing in the *Journal of Biocommunication*, proposed a revision of the Spencer and Schiffer list of descriptive cataloging elements geared to the producer of AVs rather than to the librarian familiar with the *Anglo-American Cataloging Rules*.

Efforts of NLM's AVLINE cataloging-in-publication (CIP) program, initiated on an experimental basis in February 1978, have given needed impetus to and provided leadership in this problem area;[5] NLM has sponsored CIP workshops for audiovisual producers with the cooperation of HeSCA. The objectives of the workshops were to explain existing bibliographic control problems to the media producers and to recruit the producers into the CIP program. The National Library of Medicine has agreed to catalog nonprint media from pre-release information supplied by producers and to supply a typed catalog card to the producer for incorporation onto the media before it is released for distribution.[6] Since 1979, the CIP program has been available for all instructional materials falling within the scope of AVLINE.[7] It is hoped that these developments will lead to an improved bibliographic control of media and eventually to a national bibliography of AVs in the health sciences.

SOFTWARE REFERENCE SOURCES

Information about available software appears first in the brochures or catalogs of the producers or distributors of health science media. These AV catalogs are analogous to the catalogs and brochures of book publishers and form the primary AV reference source. These catalogs are important because AV reference tools may provide insufficient information on which to make a judgment regarding acquisition, even though the information contained in these producer and distributor catalogs is the basis for the data that subsequently appear in nearly all of the existing reference tools. The National Library of Medicine's AVLINE data base and the publications derived from it are one exception: data for AVLINE are taken directly from the original media if available, the only exception being CIP items, for which producer-supplied data is used.

Software reference sources may be divided into three distinct types: (1) program indexes, (2) subject access to producer and distributor catalogs, and (3) software evaluation sources.

Program Indexes

Program indexes provide subject access to the individual programs available from producers and distributors. Typical reference questions for which program indexes are especially useful are those in which a patron requests media on a specific topic such as 16mm films on open-heart surgery or filmstrips on urinary catheterization. This type of request lends itself very well to indexes that provide a specific subject approach, such as the NLM's indexes derived from the AVLINE data base. Broad subject requests, such as one for a listing of "any available videocassettes on heart diseases," are more effectively handled on an online system. Another typical reference request requires the identification or verification of a specific media title. Program indexes that contain a name/title section are perfect for this type of reference request, provided that the patron-supplied title is correct.

The program indexes described in this chapter are current, major, multisource program indexes likely to be found in many hospital and medical libraries. Collections of individual libraries or media centers such as the Armed Forces Institute of Pathology[8] or collections of library systems such as the union list of AVs for the Veterans Administration libraries[9] have been excluded. The AVs included in such collections often have been obtained from the same producers or distributors included in the major multisource program indexes. At present these program indexes do not replace a collection of producer and distributor catalogs, but do provide subject access to a large percentage of available software in the health sciences. The lack of specific information in most of the AV program indexes, especially ordering information, reinforces the need to provide a collection of software catalogs as well.

The most important program indexes, from a bibliographic point of view, are those published by NLM from the AVLINE data base.

    11.1 AVLINE. *Audio Visuals On-LINE*. Bethesda, MD, National
    Library of Medicine.

AVLINE is a computerized data base maintained at NLM in collaboration with the Association of American Medical Colleges; NLM is
responsible for identifying, acquiring, and supplying bibliographic
descriptions for the citations in AVLINE and for providing online
access through its ELHILL retrieval programs. The Association of
American Medical Colleges (AAMC) oversees a peer review process
in which many of the AVs identified by NLM are reviewed by at least
two subject experts from a panel of 1,400 identified by the AAMC at
academic health centers throughout the country. These experts con-
tribute review data related to a program's educational design, audience level, and usefulness, and write a critical review of each item.
The AVLINE data base and the publications derived from it provide
access to more than 8,000 health science AVs in all discipline areas.

    The NLM publications are very important bibliographically be-
cause of their review data and abstracts, as well as the complete and
standardized cataloging available. Thus, the current NLM AV index
is meant not only to be a useful reference tool but also a source of
complete and accurate cataloging copy. There are three computer-
produced publications derived from the AVLINE data base:

    11.2 *National Library of Medicine Audiovisuals Catalog*. Bethesda,
    MD, 1977– .
    11.3 *National Library of Medicine AVLINE Catalog, 1975–1976*. Be-
    thesda, MD.
    11.4 *National Medical Audiovisual Center Catalog: Audiovisuals for
    the Health Sciences*. Atlanta, GA, 1974.

The current NLM *Audiovisuals Catalog* is published in three quarterly issues with an annual cumulation in lieu of the fourth quarterly
issue. Audiovisuals cataloged for this publication are listed by *Medical
Subject Headings (MeSH)* and name/title. In addition, there is a procurement source section providing the name, address, and telephone
number of the media producers and/or distributors listed in the index.
Review data and abstracts are carried in the name/title section for
many entries. A sample entry from the name/title section appears in
figure 11-2.

Figure 11-2. Sample entry from the NLM *Audiovisuals Catalog*

Edema. [Slide] / American Physiological Society. --
 [Rockville, Md.] : The Society ; [New York : for sale
 by Audio/Visual Medicine], c1976. 73 slides : col. ;
 2x2 in. & cassette (2-track. mono. 20 min.) and guide.
 -- (Illustrated lectures in renal pathophysiology) Sound
 accompaniment compatible for manual and automatic
 operation. Audience level: --Medical: undergraduate;
 graduate; continuing education. --Specialty: internal
 medicine, surgery, nephrology, pediatrics. Rating:
 Recommended. Review date: Oct. 1977. Reviewer:
 AAMC Learning method: Self instructional. Credits:
 Cecil H. Coggins.
 1. Edema – slides   I. Coggins, Cecil H. 1902–
 II. American Physiological Society (Founded 1887).
 III. Series: Illustrated lectures in renal pathophysiology
 [Slide]
 04NLM: WD 220 SC no.4.1 1976
 Abstract:
 (Critical) The superb presentation on edema clearly
 defines the pathophysiological problem and clearly
 discusses diagnosis, etiology and current treatment.
 many clinical examples are given. Unfortunately,
 diuretic therapy is only referenced, not discussed.
 Each new area of cardiovascular, hepatic and renal
 function in the genesis of edema is presented so well
 that a person with limited familiarity with these areas
 is not lost by their inclusion. Clearly, this program
 can stand alone as a teaching tool. It is highly
 recommended.
 Price:
    Sale: 65.00 (no. 903)
 Source:
    Audio/Visual Medicine   Cit. No. 7604028

**This sample citation from the name/title section has
full bibliographic information, review data, and ordering information. The subject section entry for this title
would not carry the abstract.**

The *National Library of Medicine AVLINE Catalog* lists audiovisual items cataloged by NLM from November 1975 through December 1976 for the AVLINE data base. All items in this catalog have been professionally (peer) reviewed by either AAMC or the American Association of Dental Schools (AADS) for technical quality, currency, educational design, and accuracy. Programs are listed under subject only, with no name/title section as in the previously described NLM *Audiovisuals Catalog*. Access to titles and names, including any added entries, is available online but not in the printed publication. Full bibliographic information is provided, but abstracts are excluded and available only online. There is a procurement source section.

The final product generated from the AVLINE data base is the *National Medical Audiovisual Center Catalog*. This catalog lists motion pictures and videocassettes available on short-term loan from the National Medical Audiovisual Center (NMAC) at NLM. All entries in the NMAC *Catalog* are duplicated in other publications generated from AVLINE. All materials have been peer reviewed by the AAMC or AADS and are listed by subject and name/title. The full entry appears in the name/title section. A brief listing, excluding the abstract and tracings, appears in the subject section. The motion pictures and videocassettes listed are loaned, for educational use only, to health sciences professionals, but requests for loans are not accepted from the lay public.

Peer-reviewed AVs in the NLM publications have a rating of either "recommended" or "highly recommended." Peer-reviewed AVs that are not recommended do not appear in the NLM AV indexes, although these items are maintained in the AVLINE data base. Beginning in 1977, AV materials cataloged by NLM were further categorized into two groups on the basis of content and educational design criteria.[10] Materials representing documentation of scheduled educational events such as lectures and grand rounds were processed through an abbreviated procedure and added to AVLINE without a reviewer-supplied abstract or review data. Materials that are not mere recordings of educational events continue to be funneled through the review procedure and contain review data and a reviewer-supplied abstract.

The NLM *Audiovisuals Catalog*, beginning with the 1977 cumulation, contains peer-reviewed items as well as items that have not gone through peer review for reasons other than the lecture category distinction. This latter group will not have a rating of "recommended" in the name/title section of the NLM *Audiovisuals Catalog*. Some of the items not containing the "recommended" rating may eventually go through peer review, following an anticipated content revision by the producer. Cataloging data and frequently a producer-supplied abstract are carried with these entries. Other items are lecture materials that are not candidates for peer review. Cataloging data are available for these AVs without review data or abstract. Programs that have been peer-reviewed and are *not* recommended are maintained in AVLINE, but do not appear in the printed publications generated from the data base.

Medical Subject Headings (MeSH) is the standard list of subject headings used in the printed publications of the National Library of Medicine and for subject access through the card catalogs of many medical libraries in the United States. The following AV reference tools also use *MeSH* for subject access, but unlike many of the entries in the publications derived from AVLINE, AVs included in the following tools are not, for the most part, peer-reviewed.

11.5   *Health Sciences AV Resources List: 1978–1979.* 2d ed. Farmington, CT, University of Connecticut Health Center Library, Learning Resources Center, 1978.

11.6   *Index to Audiovisual Serials in the Health Sciences.* Chicago, IL, Medical Library Association. Vol. 1– , 1977– .

11.7   *Medical Audiovisuals: A Comprehensive Catalog.* Baltimore, MD, Johns Hopkins University, Welch Medical Library Audiovisual Division, 1977.

11.8   *Selected Audiovisuals on Mental Health.* Rockville, MD, National Institute of Mental Health, National Clearinghouse of Mental Health Information, 1975.

11.9   *8MM Films in Medicine and Health Sciences.* 3d ed. Omaha, NE, University of Nebraska Medical Center, Biomedical Communications Division, 1977.

11.10 *Videolog.* New York, NY, Esselte Video. 1979– . Annual.

The *Health Sciences AV Resources List* is published in three volumes and contains approximately 10,000 titles with subject access by *MeSH*. A directory of producers and distributors and the subject index are contained in volume 1, and an alphabetic title index in volumes 2 and 3. The subject index entries are brief listings and include title, format, audience level, and year of production. Full bibliographic information, including an abstract and procurement source, is provided in the alphabetical title index. The publication lists productions from approximately 400 producers and distributors of health science media for professional continuing education, in-service training, professional undergraduate education, and patient education.

The Medical Library Association began sponsorship of the quarterly *Index to Audiovisual Serials in the Health Sciences* in 1977. The *Index* is a MEDLARS-generated tool distinct from the AV reference tools derived from the AVLINE data base. Audiotape serials, such as the productions from Audio Digest Foundation, and videotape serials, such as the productions from the Network for Continuing Medical Education (indexed since 1978), which have been peer-reviewed by the AAMC, are indexed by NLM to produce three quarterly issues and one annual cumulation. Thirty-one serial AVs are presently covered by the *Index*. Bibliographic information includes title, author, serial AV title abbreviation, volume number, issue, side of audiotape, length of presentation, and date of issue. Subject access is by *MeSH*. Several citations from the subject section of the *Index* appear in figure 11-3.

Figure 11-3. *Index to Audiovisual Serials in the Health Sciences:* sample entries

SUBJECT HEADING————————OTITIS MEDIA
Otitis media. Boles R. Audio Dig Otorhinolaryngol 23(5):Sides————VOLUME
A & B, ca. 22 min., 8 Mar 77
CROSS REFERENCE————————OVARIAN INTERSTITIAL CELLS see under OVARY

OVARY
AUDIOVISUAL TITLE————————New concepts in clinical endocrinology: influence of psycho-————SENIOR AUTHOR
pharmacologic drugs on ovarian function. Rakoff AE.
TITLE ABBREVIATION————————Audio Dig Intern Med 24(1):Side A, 18 min., 5 Jan 77————ISSUE
The future function and fortune of ovarian tissues retained in————LENGTH OF TIME
vivo during hysterectomy. Ranney B, et al.
Audio Dig Obstet Gynecol 24(8):Side B, 24 min.; Panel
DATE OF ISSUE————————Discussion, 19 Apr 77————AUDIOTAPE SIDE
OVIDUCTS, MAMMALIAN see FALLOPIAN TUBES

The first edition of *Medical Audiovisuals: A Comprehensive Catalog* appeared in 1977 with more than 5,000 entries. The bibliographic information includes title, production date, physical description, producer or distributor, format, purchase or loan information, and short summary. The main body of the *Catalog* is the subject index, arranged alphabetically by *MeSH* heading and followed by a source address index of approximately 100 producers and distributors of health science media. All formats, disciplines, and professional audience levels are included, along with patient education materials. No title or name approach is provided.

The National Institute of Mental Health, through its National Clearinghouse for Mental Health Information, has published descriptions of approximately 2,300 nonprint items in *Selected Audiovisuals on Mental Health*. Entries are arranged alphabetically by title under broad mental health topics, e.g., personality, schizophrenia, etc. Bibliographic information includes procurement source and address, price, physical description, production date, and abstract. Three sections complete the index: (1) sources for free social welfare films, (2) sources for low-cost film rental, and (3) commercial rental libraries.

The third edition of *8MM Films in Medicine and Health Sciences*, which contains 3,850 titles, was published in 1977 with grant support from NLM. The first 8mm film catalog appeared in 1969. Full bibliographic information, including a summary, appears with each entry in the alphabetical subject index, preceded by a list of subject headings (modified *MeSH*) and followed by a title index. A useful feature of the publication is the indication of the availability of a particular title in another format such as 16mm or videocassette. A distributor list of approximately 120 companies and institutions follows the title index. A report of a survey of 8mm film availability and use in the health sciences and an annotated bibliography of articles on the 8mm film format completes the catalog.[11] All subjects and disciplines and both lay and professional AVs are included.

The *Videolog* was first published in 1977 as the *Health Sciences Video Directory*. The 1979 edition contains more than 7,000 programs and series representing 150 producers and distributors of video programs. The publication is specifically aimed at health professionals, but patient education programs are also included. Subject access is via *MeSH*, and bibliographic elements include title, summary, physical description, audience, production date, and producer. A listing of producers and distributors by key names used in the body of the work, plus a listing of producers and distributors by full name with address, contact person, and telephone number, are included in separate sections of the Directory.

Four additional program indexes provide access to health science AVs by a variety of subject schemes.

11.11 *Library of Congress Catalogs: Films and Other Materials for Projection*. Washington, DC, Library of Congress. 1973– .

11.12 *Index to Health and Safety Education*. 3d ed. Los Angeles, CA, National Information Center for Educational Media, 1977.

11.13 Sequin, Marilyn, ed. *Nursing Media Index: 16MM Films*. 2d ed. Toronto, Mission Press, 1974.

11.14 *A Reference List of Audiovisual Materials Produced by the United States Government, 1978*. Washington, DC, National Audiovisual Center, 1978.

Library of Congress subject headings are used in *Films and Other Materials for Projection*, which is a subject and name/title index to media cataloged by the Library of Congress. The publication is produced quarterly, with annual and quinquennial cumulations. The Library of Congress (LC) attempts to catalog all media released in the United States or Canada that have educational or instructional value. Videocassettes listed are limited to those distributed by the National

Audiovisual Center. Data for the catalog entries are supplied from producers, manufacturers, film libraries, or distributing agencies. The National Audiovisual Center provides the information for United States government materials. Prior to 1972, LC cataloged all copyrighted works (1951–57) or copyrighted work added to its collection (1957–71), but no restrictions of this sort presently exist. There is a brief listing of the media in the subject section, with full cataloging following *Anglo-American Cataloging Rules* and including a summary in the name/title section. A directory of producers and distributors for the cataloged items appeared from 1973 to 1975. The audience level is indicated when available. Older items cataloged by LC appear in *Library of Congress Catalog. Motion Pictures and Filmstrips.* [12]

The *Index to Health and Safety Education* is one of several indexes published by the National Information Center for Educational Media (NICEM) at the University of Southern California in Los Angeles. The third edition (1977) contains more than 33,000 entries representing eight different media formats. A cooperative arrangement allows NICEM to obtain data supplied to LC by producers and distributors of media. Data supplied by LC are identified in the NICEM index entries by the presence of LC card numbers. The *Index* is generated from a computerized data base maintained by NICEM and is available online through Lockheed Information Systems' DIALOG retrieval programs. The *Index* is divided into three sections: (1) a subject guide by broad subject with a listing of media titles; (2) an alphabetical section by title, listing summaries, physical descriptions, formats, producers, and distributors; (3) a directory of producers and distributors. Much of the information in the *Index* is in a coded format with an explanation for the codes provided in an introductory section. The subject guide section is preceded by a subject heading outline, which is essential to consult when a subject search of the *Index* is required. The subject guide is organized alphabetically by broad subject (e.g., Science-Natural), subdivided alphabetically by specific area (e.g., Biology, Physiology [Human]-Heart and Circulation) and within specific area subdivided further by media format. Occasionally, the subject approach is too broad. "Medicine," a subject heading classified under "Health and Safety," occupies 19 pages and covers nearly 7,000 individual titles.

The *Nursing Media Index: 16MM Films* was published as a second edition in 1974. Approximately 1,000 titles are indexed by broad subject, and bibliographic information includes a summary, physical description, and distributor. Procurement sources are mostly Canadian, with a few from the United States; many, however, are Canadian offices of United States firms.

The National Audiovisual Center (NAC) in Washington, DC, maintains a master data file of approximately 10,000 citations to AVs for sale or rent. The NAC was created in 1969 to distribute AVs produced by or for the various agencies, branches, and bureaus of the United States government, and it serves as a clearinghouse of all federal audiovisual materials. Materials from NAC are identified in several printed select lists in various disciplines such as medicine and dentistry and in a monthly publication entitled *Select List*, which lists all subjects added to the NAC data base. The major printed catalog of NAC is *A Reference List of Audiovisual Materials Produced by the United States Government, 1978*. It lists more than 6,000 AV programs selected from more than 10,000 programs maintained on the master data file. The publication contains an outline of subject headings used, a subject index, and a title index. Sale and rental prices are listed in a separate price list section by unique order number found with the full entry for each citation in the title index. Full names of sponsoring or producing agencies, which appear in coded format in the title index, are listed separately in a sponsor and producer code list. Bibliographic information in the title index includes physical description, producing and sponsoring organization, NAC order number, sale/rental availability, series note, and summary. All printed publications are available free of charge from NAC, and telephone and mail reference inquiries are accepted by the NAC Reference Section.

Subject Access to Producers and Distributors

Another method of locating relevant software is through the use of reference tools that provide subject access to producers and distributors. These tools list names, addresses, subject area, and formats of various producers or distributors instead of individual media programs. The assumption is that one has access to a collection of software catalogs that must be consulted to identify individual media programs. Specific subject requests for media or requests to identify specific titles will still be more efficiently handled by program indexes, but broad subject requests can be handled effectively by tools that provide subject access to producers and distributors. Program indexes seem inherently better, but given the present state of AV bibliographic control (or lack thereof) the following publications are useful.

11.15 *AVMP: Audiovisual Market Place; A Multimedia Guide.* New York, NY, Bowker, 1969– . Annual.

11.16 Ash, Joan, and Stevenson, Michael. *Health; A Multimedia Source Guide.* New York, NY, Bowker, 1976.

11.17 *AV Source Directory. A Subject Index to Health Science AV Producer/Distributor Catalogs.* Edited by Bruce Ardis. Compiled by the Audiovisual Subcommittee of the Midwest Health Science Library Network. Chicago, IL, Midwest Health Science Library Network, John Crerar Library, 1977.

11.18 *Directory of Spoken Voice Audio-Cassettes.* Los Angeles, CA, Cassette Information Services, 1976.

11.19 Martyn, Dorian E., Spencer, Dorothy A., and Duke, Phyllis M. *Source List for Patient Education Material.* Millbrae, CA, Health Sciences Communications Association, 1978.

The *Audiovisual Market Place* is an important general AV reference tool, published annually, which includes information on both AV software and hardware. Software information includes subject access to producers and distributors. Unfortunately, the subject access is so broad (e.g., the headings "Medicine" or "Science") that the tool is almost useless from a subject standpoint. It is quite useful, however, for verification of addresses, telephone numbers, and production characteristics. The "Reference Books and Directories" section of this publication is invaluable. Additional software information includes production companies classified by media and subject; production services such as laboratory and sound recording services; a listing of public radio and TV program libraries that lend, rent, or sell their productions; and a listing of AV cataloging services.

A more useful tool, in terms of specific subject access to producers and distributors, is *Health: A Multimedia Source Guide.* This is an annotated list of organizations that deal with health-related matters, including publishers, AV producers and distributors, libraries, and government agencies. The AV producer and distributor section includes 188 producers and distributors, listed alphabetically by name. Organizations that produce or distribute AVs but are described in other sections of the *Guide* are cross-referenced in the AV section. Each entry includes the name, address, telephone number, purpose, special services, and publications of the organization. There is a general organization index, an index to agencies providing free or inexpensive material, and a subject index.

The *AV Source Directory* is the most comprehensive listing of AV producers and distributors available. Published in 1977, it contains descriptions of more than 600 producers and distributors of health science media. Bibliographic information includes name, address, telephone number, media format, distribution method (e.g., purchase, loan, rent), approximate number of AVs available, and a list of *MeSH* headings to indicate subject scope. Entries are listed alphabetically by name with *MeSH* subject indexes by discipline to provide broad subject access and by specific *MeSH* headings to provide specific subject access. The scope of the catalog is very broad. The compilers tried to identify all producers and distributors having audiovisuals for use by health sciences professionals. Numerous agencies listed under "Health Education" and various patient terms in the subject index indicate that the subject area of patient education was not excluded from the index. The comprehensive nature and relative currency of the *Directory* qualifies it as an index to even the largest of producer and distributor catalog collections.

A directory that provides subject access to producers and distributors in a specific media format is the *Directory of Spoken Voice Audio-Cassettes*. The *Directory*, which is an alphabetical listing of audiocassette producers with a description of their programs, is limited in scope to programs aimed at the adult or college level. The index to the publication is a dictionary index of broad subjects and major program titles. Entries include both serial and monographic audiocassettes.

The need to locate media for patient education has received much attention recently, at least in part because of a stress on informed consent and the consumer rights movement. These issues and others have created the impetus to provide patient education materials in the health care setting. The federal agency concerned with patient education, the Bureau of Health Education, provides a bibliography of patient education resource materials upon request.[13] The most useful publication in the subject area of patient education is the *Source List for Patient Education Materials*, published by the Health Science Communication Association in 1978. The *Source List* provides access to 580 print and nonprint sources of patient education materials, listed alphabetically by name. There is a *MeSH* subject index.

The following are journals that review audiovisuals. It should be noted that AV reviews may not always be a regular feature in all of the journals.

1. ACCEL, *Audio Tape Journal in Cardiology* (American College of Cardiology Extended Learning)
2. *AHIL Quarterly* (Association of Hospital and Institutional Libraries)
3. *American Family Physician*
4. *American Journal of Nursing*
5. *American Rehabilitation*
6. *Biomedical Communications*
7. *British Medicine*
8. *Community Mental Health Journal*
9. *The Dental Assistant*
10. *Health Education/Education Sanitaire*
11. *Hospital and Community Psychiatry*
12. *Hospital Topics*
13. *Journal of the American Medical Association*
14. *Journal of the American Dietetic Association*
15. *Journal of Audiovisual Media in Medicine*
16. *Journal of Biocommunication*
17. *Journal of Family Practice*
18. *Journal of Nursing Administration*
19. *Journal of Nutrition Education*
20. *Journal of Sex and Marital Therapy*
21. *Mental Hygiene*
22. *MLA News ("Media Notes"),* Medical Library Association
23. *Nursing Outlook*
24. *Occupational Health Nursing*
25. *The Physiologist* (v. 18, no. 4, November 1975 supplement and other issues)
26. *Postgraduate Medicine*
27. *The Practitioner*
28. *Previews*
29. *RC; Respiratory Care*

Figure 11-4. List of journals providing reviews of AV media

Software Evaluation

Given the differences in teaching methods between one institution and another, it is not surprising that most institutions prefer to preview and evaluate media prior to purchase. The need to evaluate becomes increasingly important as media and equipment become more and more expensive. A good media review can save time and money by indicating the material's appropriateness in a well-written summary or abstract. A number of journals provide reviews of media productions (figure 11-4), along with the AVLINE data base and the publications derived from it. The following is an example of a specialized evaluation tool for health sciences AVs:

11.20 *Hospital/Health Care Training Media Profiles.* New York, NY, Olympic Media Information. Vol. 1– , 1974– .

Reviews written for *Hospital/Health Care Training Media Profiles* come mainly from the subscribers themselves and include synopses that describe in program sequence the story elements of the programs. The evaluation section for each review is distinct from the synopsis or summary and will include a recommendation on the use of the material and, when appropriate, any negative statements about the value of the program. Other bibliographic elements include title, series title, physical description, audience, accompanying materials, and procurement source. The publication provides title and *MeSH* subject indexes plus a format index that gives access to reviews by media format. *Profiles* is currently published bimonthly in looseleaf format. A cumulative index exists for the first three complete volumes. Subject emphasis is on hospital and health care training as opposed to medical, dental, and nursing education.

HARDWARE REFERENCE SOURCES

Sources of information regarding the equipment on which media are used or carrels in which equipment is housed can be divided into sources that evaluate hardware and sources that only provide access to manufacturers and dealers of hardware. The annual *Audiovisual Market Place,* mentioned previously, falls into the latter classification. Equipment manufacturers are listed alphabetically by firm name, with a classified index by equipment type. Information for each firm includes name, address, telephone number, type of product manufactured and, in many cases, the sales or marketing manager. Equipment dealers are listed alphabetically within each state. Other sources of information regarding equipment include:

11.21 *Audio-Visual Equipment Directory.* Fairfax, VA, National Audio-Visual Association. 1955– . Annual.

11.22 *Library Technology Reports.* Chicago, IL, American Library Association. Vol. 1– , 1965– .

11.23 *Sourcebook of Library Technology.* Chicago, IL, American Library Association, 1978.

11.24 *EPIE Report.* New York, NY, Educational Products Information Exchange Institute. Vol. 1– , 1967– .

11.25 *Annotated Directory of Parts and Services for Audiovisual Equipment 1976–1977.* EPIE Report No. 75. New York, NY, Educational Products Information Exchange Institute, 1977.

The *Audio-Visual Equipment Directory* is an annual publication of the National Audio-Visual Association (NAVA), which, however, does not evaluate the equipment listed in the *Directory*, stating that the inclusion of equipment does not imply endorsement and omission does not imply disapproval. The *Directory* includes both domestic- and foreign-manufactured equipment available in North America. Information on items listed is contributed by the manufacturers. Entries are classified by type of equipment and then arranged alphabetically by proprietary name. A photograph of each piece of equipment described is a useful feature. Other pertinent information includes model number, price, physical description, accessories, and notes indicating special features, available modifications, or ordering specifics. An index to contributors provides access to the names and addresses of the manufacturers of featured AV equipment. Special features of the *Directory* are an alphabetical product index by trade name; a directory of AV dealers, film libraries, and consulting companies arranged by state with coded information of products and services; and special charts and tables on screen size, typical running times of films, etc.

Library Technology Reports (LTR) is a bimonthly publication of the American Library Association (ALA). From the introduction: "[LTR] provides critical evaluations of products and systems used in libraries, media centers, schools, and other educational institutions. These evaluations are designed to enable management and staff of these institutions to make efficient and economical purchasing decisions." Evaluated items, not all of which are related to AVs, are chosen on the basis of interest to subscribers of *LTR* and the availability of standards and effective evaluative methods and procedures. Generally there is a photograph of each evaluated item.

These evaluations have been compiled on microfiche in the *Sourcebook of Library Technology*. The 1978 edition of the *Sourcebook* is an edited compilation of evaluative material previously published in *LTR* from 1965 to 1977. A printed table of contents and a detailed index facilitate the use of the microfiche compilation.

Test programs and procedures for items reported in the *LTR* and *Sourcebook* are developed by ALA in consultation with nationally recognized independent labs. One such testing organization is the Educational Products Information Exchange Institute (EPIE Institute). The EPIE Institute was chartered in 1967 as a nonprofit consumer-supported agency by the Regents of the University of the State of

New York. The Institute compiles and disseminates information about instructional materials (e.g., basic science textbooks for high schools); equipment, including AV equipment; and systems. Income for EPIE is derived from membership and from subscriptions to its semi-monthly consumer-oriented newsletters, *EPIEgram* and *Performance*. The Institute publishes a number of reports each year; EPIE Report No. 75, the *Annotated Directory of Parts and Services for Audiovisual Equipment 1976–77*, is especially noteworthy. The *Directory* was developed by the Association of Audio-Visual Technicians and is divided into two sections. A brand-name section provides references to one or more manufacturers or dealers in the manufacturer/dealer section who can supply parts, servicing information, or publications about the brand cited. The manufacturer/dealer listing provides the address, telephone number, contact persons, specific ordering information, available service manuals, and other pertinent information if applicable. Other EPIE numbered reports evaluate 16mm projectors, filmstrip projectors, and the like.

In brief, a reference tool such as the *Audiovisual Market Place* is very useful for verifying address information of equipment manufacturers or dealers or for compiling a list of manufacturers of specific types of hardware. However, to find out which equipment is currently available, the specifications of the equipment, price, ordering information, and a photograph, the *Audio-Visual Equipment Directory* is the more appropriate tool. The evaluation of specific types of hardware for use in educational institutions is provided by the *Library Technology Reports* and by the *EPIE Report* series.

REFERENCES

[1] McIlvaine, Paul M., and Brantz, Malcolm H. Audiovisual Materials: A Survey of Bibliographic Controls in Distributors' Catalogs. *Bull. Med. Libr. Assoc.* 65: 17–21, Jan. 1977.

[2] Spencer, Dorothy, and Schiffer, Pamela. List of Descriptive Cataloging Elements for Use in Bibliographic Control of Non-print Materials. *J. of Biocommun.* 4: 18–32, 1977.

[3] American Library Association, Canadian Library Association, and the Library Association (London). *Anglo-American Cataloging Rules, Chapter 12.* Revised ed. Chicago, IL, American Library Association, 1975.

[4]Bogen, Betty. Guidelines for Producers and Distributors of Media for the Health Sciences. *J. of Biocommun.* 4: 24–29, 1977.

[5]CIP Workshop for Audiovisuals. *NLM News.* 33: 3–4, Mar. 1978.

[6]White, Virginia. AVLINE Update. *NLM Tech. Bull.* No. 106: 17, Feb. 1978.

[7]HeSCA/NLM CIP Project Update. *NLM News.* 33: 3, Dec. 1978.

[8]Armed Forces Institute of Pathology. *Medical Films and Related Audiovisual Aids.* Washington, DC, 1977.

[9]*Union List of Audiovisuals in the Library Network of the Veterans Administration.* Washington, DC, Veterans Administration, 1976.

[10]Schoolman, Harold. AVLINE Status Report. *NLM Tech. Bull.* No. 99: 8, Jul. 1977.

[11]Benschoter, Reba Ann. "Survey Update; 8MM Film Availability and Use in Health Sciences." In: *8MM Films in Medicine and Health Sciences.* 3rd ed. Omaha, NE, University of Nebraska Medical Center, Biomedical Communications Division, 1977.

[12]*Library of Congress Catalog. Motion Pictures and Filmstrips.* 1953–1972, Washington, DC, Library of Congress. 1953–57, v. 28 of *The National Union Catalog* (1953–57); 1958–62, v. 53 of *The National Union Catalog* (1958–62); 1963–67, v. 2 of *The National Union Catalog* (1963–67); 1968–72, v. 4 of *The National Union Catalog* (1968–72).

[13]*Current Resources in Patient Education.* Atlanta, GA, U.S. Department of Health, Education, and Welfare. Public Health Service, Center for Disease Control, Bureau of Health Education, Community Program Development Division, n.d.

READINGS

Fenske, Ruth. Audiovisual Services. In: *Basic Library Management for Health Science Librarians.* Section N. Rev. ed. Chicago, IL, Midwest Health Science Library Network, 1975. pp. N-1–N-31.

Homan, J. Michael. *CE 31: Basic Media Management-Software.* Chicago, IL, Medical Library Association, 1979.

Hunter, George H. *Establishing a Learning Resource Center in a Medical Library.* Atlanta, GA, National Medical Audiovisual Center, 1974.

Laird, Dugan. *A User's Look at the Audio-visual World.* Fairfax, VA, National Audiovisual Association, 1974.

Moreland, Ernest F., and Craig, James F. *Developing a Learning Resource Center: A Guide to Organizing a Learning Resource Center in Health Science Educational Institutions.* Atlanta, GA, National Medical Audiovisual Center, 1974.

Strohlein, Alfred. *The Management of 35MM Medical Slides.* New York, NY, United Business Publications, Inc., 1975.

Weinsieder, Gail, et al. The Development of Audiovisual Resources in Hospital Information Centers. In: Bloomquist, Harold, ed., *Library Practice in Hospitals; A Basic Guide.* Cleveland, OH, Case Western Reserve, 1972. pp. 193–217.

CHAPTER 12

Medical
and
Health Statistics

REBECCA W. DAVIDSON and RICHARD E. HINSON

Medical and health statistics encompass a highly interdisciplinary area of medical reference and represent challenges to the librarian that may well be unique in the field. Rarely will one find such an array of reference tools at one's disposal, coupled with such opportunities for frustration. Today's medical reference librarian can characterize the most obscure syndrome, provide toxicity data for a list of compounds that seems to grow exponentially, and sometimes even map a chromosome. Yet the same librarian may be forced into a posture of defeat when asked to produce a seemingly obvious statistic.

Difficulties with statistics stem more from problems of access, consistency, and timeliness than from a shortage of good reference materials. The multiplicity of numbers that can appear in one table of statistics, for example, necessarily limits subject access to relatively large categories. Library patrons, on the other hand, often require specifics. Variations in coverage—geographical areas, time periods, methods of data collection and analysis, sample size, and definitions of categories—occur like the plague. Users, however, expect consistent reporting and reliable comparisons. Finally, most statistics are out of date long before they hit the printed page.

All of the above would be inconsequential were it not for the importance of health-related statistics and the demands placed upon them. Such statistics exist in the first place to provide planners, administrators, and researchers with a comprehensive picture of the nation's health. Statistics can be used to shed light on various aspects of the population, to understand how health services and health programs are being utilized, to evaluate the effectiveness of health care delivery, and to identify the country's health care needs.

Health-related statistics have recently become even more sought after with the emergence of health care as a major political issue. Careful evaluation of such questions now before the public depends in part on the availability and accessibility of statistics. The national debates on hospital cost containment, aging, and national health insurance, for example, hinge by and large on statistical proof. As adherents of the various options use statistics to buttress their opinions, information resources, such as libraries and librarians, fall under additional pressure to provide accurate data to both the specialist and the citizenry at large.

Health-related statistics include a wide spectrum of information—from population size, to incidence of disease, to physicians' incomes. For purposes of clarification, statistical data can be divided into two broad overlapping categories: (1) *Vital and demographic statistics* are used to define and characterize a population. They include statistics about births, deaths, marriages, divorces, the occurrence of illness and injury, and the size, density, and migration of the population. (2) *Socioeconomic statistics*, on the other hand, define and characterize the health care industry. These comprise, among other things, the availability and distribution of health manpower, the utilization of health resources and facilities, and expenditures for health care.

Socioeconomic and demographic statistics are often correlated in the hope of discovering cause and effect. The incidence of disease in a certain area, for example, may be compared to the distribution of primary care physicians in the same region. The two-part division, however, can serve as a useful heuristic model in determining where to find an answer.

USEFUL TERMINOLOGY

Although the jargon of health statistics is certainly more accessible than that of many other areas of medical reference, a few terms need to be defined. All definitions are taken from *A Discursive Dictionary of Health Care*,[1] a useful reference source in its own right:

acute disease: a disease which is characterized by a single episode of a fairly short duration from which the patient returns to his normal or previous state and level of activity.

chronic diseases: diseases which have one or more of the following characteristics: are permanent; leave residual disability; are caused by non-reversible pathological alteration; require special training of the patient for rehabilitation; or may be expected to require a long period of supervision, observation, or care.

health facilities: buildings, including physical plant, equipment, and supplies, used in providing health services. They are one major type of health resource and include hospitals, nursing homes, and ambulatory care centers. Usually they are not intended to include the offices of individual practitioners.

health manpower: collectively, all men and women working in the provision of health services whether as individual practitioners or employees of health institutions and programs; whether or not professionally trained; and whether or not subject to public regulation. Facilities and manpower are the principal health resources used in producing health services.

health resources: resources (human, monetary, or material) used in producing health care and services. They include money, health manpower, health facilities, equipment, and supplies. Resources, available or used, can be measured and described for an area, population, or an individual program or service.

incidence: in epidemiology, the number of cases of disease, infection, or some other event having their *onset* during a prescribed period of time in relation to the unit of population in which they occur. It measures morbidity or other events as they happen *over a period of time*. Compare with *prevalence*.

morbidity: the extent of illness, injury, or disability in a defined population. It is usually expressed in general or specific rates of incidence or prevalence. Sometimes used to refer to any episode of disease.

mortality: death. Used to describe the relation of deaths to the population in which they occur. The mortality rate (death rate) expresses the number of deaths in a unit of population within a prescribed time and may be expressed as crude death rates (e.g., total deaths in relation to total population during a year) or as rates specific for diseases and, sometimes, for age, sex, or other attributes (e.g., number of deaths from cancer in white males in relation to the white male population during a year).

notifiable: applied to a disease which providers are required (usually by law) to report to Federal, State or local public health officials when diagnosed (such as tuberculosis, diphtheria and syphilis). Notifiable diseases are those of public interest by reason of their infectiousness, severity, or frequency.

prevalence: the number of cases of disease, infected persons, or persons with some other attribute, *present* at a particular time and in relation to the size of the population from which drawn. It is a measurement of morbidity *at a moment in time,* for example, the number of cases of hemophilia in the country as of the first of the year. Prevalence equals incidence times average case duration.

vital statistics: statistics relating to births (natality), deaths (mortality), marriages, health and disease (morbidity).

The librarian must take special note of the implications of *incidence* and *prevalence, acute* and *chronic*: they serve to illustrate just one problem in locating statistical information on health topics. Rarely, if ever, are incidence statistics available for chronic disease. The long-term nature of chronic disease makes it difficult to determine exactly when a disease, such as alcoholism, has its *onset,* which is the primary piece of information needed for incidence statistics. People with chronic diseases, in fact, may not contact their physicians until an acute complication of the disease manifests itself. Even prevalence statistics may be difficult to locate for either acute or chronic diseases unless they are notifiable. Except for notifiable, communicable diseases, which are reportable by law to the Center for Disease Control, no agency has ongoing responsibility for collection of statistics on all diseases.

On the other hand, one of the virtues of statistical reference is the fact that many of the major producers of statistical data are easily identifiable. An awareness of what organizations these are and a familiarity with their publications can serve not only as an aid in finding an answer in a printed source, but also as a means of obtaining information that has not yet been published. Quite often a simple telephone call will provide an answer or at least put one on the right track.

AGENCIES AND ORGANIZATIONS

The primary responsibility for the collection and dissemination of medical and health statistics in the United States rests with various agencies in the Department of Health, Education, and Welfare. Organized in 1960, the National Center for Health Statistics (NCHS) "is the principal organization for providing statistical intelligence on vital events, health, injuries, illness, impairments, use of medical, dental, hospital and other health care services and on the facilities and manpower which provide these services. The central mission of NCHS is to establish and maintain a set of mechanisms that provide for producing the information necessary in these fields."[2] This description translates into an impressive amount of data, which the NCHS collects, analyzes, and disseminates to the public. This is done principally through a national vital registration system, covering births, deaths, marriages, and divorces,[3] and by a series of ongoing surveys of the ambulatory and institutionalized population and of health facilities. The Center also sponsors and conducts extensive statistical research, trains personnel both within the United States and abroad, and administers the Cooperative Health Statistics System, the last being an attempt to involve federal, state, and local governments in the coordination of statistical information. The major publications of NCHS are the *Vital Statistics of the U.S.*, the *Monthly Vital Statistics Report*, and the *Vital and Health Statistics Series*.[4]

The Center for Disease Control (CDC) protects "the public health of the Nation by providing leadership and direction in the prevention and control of diseases and other preventable conditions,"[5] including, for example, childhood lead-based paint poisoning, urban rat control, and vector-borne disease. The CDC conducts research, consultation, and training in such areas as occupational safety and health, epidemiology, and health education. Activities of the CDC "focus on the improvement of the health care system through emphasis on prevention and investigations, surveillance and control operations . . . rather than through direct treatment."[6] One of its major activities is the collection of statistics on reportable diseases. This information is published in the *Morbidity and Mortality Weekly Report*, and also sent to the World Health Organization. The CDC also publishes considerable statistical material in its national surveillance reports on specific diseases and conditions.

Although the NCHS and the CDC are the two most noticeable agencies within the federal government that collect and disseminate statistics, nearly every agency produces statistics of some kind. The National Institutes of Health, for example, conduct research in the areas of cancer, heart disease, infectious diseases, child health and development, and neurological diseases, to name a few. They can be an important source of statistical information on incidence, prevalence, and cost of treating these conditions. The Health Resources Administration and the Social Security Administration have information on the socioeconomic aspects of health care. Finally, the Bureau of the Census, although outside the Department of Health, Education, and Welfare, conducts the single most important demographic survey in the country.

A consideration of the problems with national statistics that were underscored at the beinning of this chapter, magnified one hundred-fold, yields some conception of the difficulties encountered when working with international statistics. Questions about reliability and comparability must be raised with all statistics, but particularly those produced in developing countries, where efforts are often made to present a better picture of conditions than actually exists. In some areas, for example, infant deaths are not counted if the infant is less than six months old. Organizations such as the United Nations, the Pan American Health Organization, UNESCO, and the International Labour Organization develop useful statistical data incidental to their primary purposes.

The World Health Organization (WHO), however, serves as the primary international agency in the health field. It conducts extensive programs in the treatment and prevention of diseases, the training of health personnel, and the collection and dissemination of information, including statistics. It assists countries with the development of collecting methods and also publishes the most comprehensive set of international health statistics available in the *World Health Statistics Quarterly* and the *World Health Statistics Annual.*

In addition to governmental or quasigovernmental agencies, a number of private associations exist, which are prolific producers and consumers of statistics. Voluntary and private organizations such as the American Heart Association or the Cystic Fibrosis Foundation can be important sources of statistics in their areas of interest. Suffice it to say that any association that represents an investment in the health care industry will have a statistical publication of one sort or another. Noteworthy are the American Medical Association, American Hospital Association, American Dental Association, National League for

Nursing, American Nurses Association, and Association of American Medical Colleges. These societies conduct and publish surveys of their membership or issue special studies that reveal statistical information unavailable elsewhere. For information on the cost of medical care and other aspects of health care economics, life and health insurance companies can be an excellent source of statistics. Some of the most reliable reference materials in the area of health manpower and facilities issue from the private sector.

GENERAL STRATEGY FOR LOCATING STATISTICAL INFORMATION

As with any other area of reference work, one should take a logical approach to finding the sought-after statistic. Admittedly, statistical questions are more likely to appear difficult or specialized because of the wealth of material available and the particularity of the request. There are, however, a few points to keep in mind that should make answering such questions easier.

The librarian should begin by categorizing the question as much as possible. First, what is the subject of the request? Does it fall into one of the groups already discussed; for example, is it a question about disease (morbidity) or death (mortality)? Is the disease chronic or infectious? What population is of interest? Does the question have to do with health manpower, health resources, or health care economics? Second, which of the major producers or compilers of statistical information would be likely to have these facts? Does this organization have an ongoing or special publication? The card catalog of the library may be helpful here. One could look either under the name of the organization or under the subject itself, using one of the subheadings for material that contains statistical information. If the library uses *Medical Subject Headings (MeSH)* in its card catalog, there are a number of useful subheadings under which statistical data can best be located. These subheadings include: charts, complications, etiology, manpower, mortality, occurrence, statistics, supply and distribution, tables, and utilization.[7]

Much statistical information is never compiled into a major source, but remains hidden in journal articles or government reports. Another problem with statistical data is timeliness—or lack of it. To cite only one example: the latest (in 1979) available published volume of the *Vital Statistics of the United States* contains data for 1975. One way to solve both of these problems is to use indexes and abstracts. The most useful indexes for statistical information in the health sciences are *Index Medicus, Medical Socioeconomic Research Sources,* and the *American Statistics Index.*

Using *Index Medicus,* one can often locate a relevant topic in *Medical Subject Headings.* Then one of the subheadings listed above can be searched for statistical data, with the exception of "charts," "statistics," and "tables," which may only be used in the card catalog. For finding general articles in the area of demography or vital statistics, one or more of the headings in figure 12-1 may be helpful.

Figure 12-1. *MeSH* headings in the area of demography or vital statistics

N1 — HEALTH CARE - POPULATION CHARACTERISTICS

POPULATION CHARACTERISTICS (NON MESH)

POPULATION CHARACTERISTICS (NON MESH)	N1			
DEMOGRAPHY	N1.224	I1.782.616.		
AGE FACTORS	N1.224.67	G7.168.142		
ETHNIC GROUPS	N1.224.317	I1.76.201.	I1.880.143.	M1.194
HANDICAPPED	N1.224.406	M1.289		
HEALTH SURVEYS	N1.224.458	G3.850.520.		
DENTAL HEALTH SURVEYS	N1.224.458.251	G3.890.160		
DMF INDEX	N1.224.458.251.266	G3.890.160.		
ORAL HYGIENE INDEX*	N1.224.458.251.576	G3.890.160.		
PERIODONTAL INDEX	N1.224.458.251.720	E6.721.658	G3.890.160.	
HEALTH STATUS INDICATORS*	N1.224.458.470	G3.850.520.		
MASS SCREENING	N1.224.458.527	E1.563 N2.421.726.	G3.850.520.	N2.421.143.
GENETIC SCREENING	N1.224.458.527.125	E1.563.390	G3.850.520.	N2.421.143.
MASS CHEST X-RAY	N1.224.458.527.443	E1.302.577 G3.850.520.	E1.563.443 N2.421.143.	E1.818.870. N2.421.726.
MULTIPHASIC SCREENING	N1.224.458.527.633	E1.563.633 N2.421.726.	G3.850.520.	N2.421.143.
NUTRITION SURVEYS	N1.224.458.696	G3.850.520.		
DIET SURVEYS*	N1.224.458.696.385	G3.850.520.		
MINORITY GROUPS	N1.224.593	I1.880.371	M1.403	
POPULATION	N1.224.716	I1.782.616		
POPULATION DENSITY	N1.224.716.533	I1.782.616.		
POPULATION GROWTH	N1.224.716.700	I1.782.616.		
SEX FACTORS	N1.224.816			
VITAL STATISTICS	N1.224.935			
BIRTH RATE	N1.224.935.161			
LIFE EXPECTANCY	N1.224.935.464	H1.548.832.		
MORBIDITY	N1.224.935.597			
MORTALITY	N1.224.935.698			
FETAL DEATH	N1.224.935.698.302	C13.703.243	C23.240.477	
INFANT MORTALITY	N1.224.935.698.489			

N1 — HEALTH CARE - POPULATION CHARACTERISTICS

POPULATION CHARACTERISTICS (NON MESH)
   DEMOGRAPHY
      VITAL STATISTICS
         MORTALITY
            MATERNAL MORTALITY

MATERNAL MORTALITY	N1.224.935.698.653			
SEX RATIO	N1.224.935.780	G5.414.791	G8.665.831	
HEALTH AND DISEASE (NON MESH)	N1.407			
DISEASE	N1.407.306	C23.280		
ACUTE DISEASE	N1.407.306.137	C23.280.50		
CHRONIC DISEASE	N1.407.306.350	C23.280.176		
CONVALESCENCE	N1.407.306.485	C23.280.224		
HEALTH	N1.407.540			
FAMILY HEALTH*	N1.407.540.205	I1.880.225.		
MENTAL HEALTH	N1.407.540.408	F2.418	F4.366	
ORAL HEALTH	N1.407.540.576			
PHYSICAL FITNESS	N1.407.540.730	I3.621		
RURAL HEALTH	N1.407.540.750			
URBAN HEALTH*	N1.407.540.770			
WORLD HEALTH	N1.407.540.800			
RESIDENCE CHARACTERISTICS	N1.696			
CATCHMENT AREA (HEALTH)	N1.696.100	N3.349.650.		
HOUSING	N1.696.342	G3.230.150.		
PUBLIC HOUSING	N1.696.324.631			
RESIDENTIAL MOBILITY	N1.696.596			
EMIGRATION AND IMMIGRATION	N1.696.596.321			
TRANSIENTS AND MIGRANTS	N1.696.596.797	M1.920		
RURAL POPULATION	N1.696.704			
URBAN POPULATION	N1.696.876			
SOCIOECONOMIC FACTORS	N1.824	I1.880.840		
EDUCATIONAL STATUS	N1.824.196			
EMPLOYMENT	N1.824.245			
FAMILY CHARACTERISTICS	N1.824.308	F1.829.263.	I1.880.225.	
DIVORCE	N1.824.308.266	F1.829.263.	I1.880.225.	I1.880.735.
MARRIAGE	N1.824.308.526	F1.829.263.	I1.880.225.	
SINGLE PERSON	N1.824.308.794	F1.829.263.	I1.880.225.	M1.785
INCOME	N1.824.417			
PENSIONS	N1.824.417.510			
SALARIES AND FRINGE BENEFITS	N1.824.417.700	N4.452.677.		
MEDICAL INDIGENCY	N1.824.460			
OCCUPATIONS	N1.824.547			
CAREER MOBILITY	N1.824.547.330	N4.452.677.		
POVERTY	N1.824.600	I1.880.735.	I1.880.840.	
SOCIAL CHANGE	N1.824.737	I1.880.526		
SOCIAL CLASS	N1.824.782	I1.880.552	I1.880.840.	
SOCIAL MOBILITY	N1.824.782.673	I1.880.552.	I1.880.840.	
SOCIAL CONDITIONS	N1.824.827	I1.880.578		
UNEMPLOYMENT	N1.824.925			

* INDICATES MINOR DESCRIPTOR

National Library of Medicine, *Medical Subject Headings, Tree Structures, 1979*. Springfield, VA, NTIS, 1978, pp. 410–411.

Of particular interest among the approximately 3,000 biomedical journals indexed for *Index Medicus* are the *Vital and Health Statistics* series of NCHS, the *World Health Statistics Quarterly*, the *Mental Health Statistical Note,* and the *Statistical Bulletin* of the Metropolitan Life Insurance Company.

Medical Socioeconomic Research Sources, published by the American Medical Association (see chapter 4, ref. 4.3), covers a wide range of material not accessible through *Index Medicus* or other sources, including government reports, books, journals, newspapers, and legislation. It is a very useful key to health care economics and utilization of health services. A drawback—and one that is particularly frustrating when using an index—is that it is published only quarterly with an annual cumulation and is thus more useful for recent history than for very current data.

American Statistics Index claims to be the master index to all publications of the federal government that contain statistical information. In its own words:

Specifically, the purpose of *ASI* is to perform the following functions, promptly and comprehensively:

IDENTIFY the statistical data published by all branches and agencies of the Federal Government.

CATALOG the publications in which these data appear, providing full bibliographic information about each publication.

ANNOUNCE new publications as they appear.

DESCRIBE the contents of these publications fully.

INDEX this information in full subject detail.

MICROPUBLISH virtually all the publications covered by ASI, thereby providing on a continuing basis, reliable access to the statistics themselves.[8]

As such, the *Index* is virtually the only key to ephemeral publications such as *Advance Data* and can be a useful tool in locating information in unexpected places. For periodical literature published by the federal government, *American Statistics Index* gives an open entry for the title followed by analytics of particular issues appearing during the period covered by the index. For all items covered, detailed information is provided about the nature of the data and the parameters they cover. Many points of access are provided, among them subjects, titles, agency report numbers, and such special categories as census division, by occupation or by age.

For the literature of health planning, two additional services are worthy of mention: *Abstracts of Health Care Management Studies* (see chapter 4, ref. 4.12) from the University of Michigan School of Public Health and *Weekly Government Abstracts: Health Planning* from the National Technical Information Service. Both cover published and unpublished report literature, and both provide document delivery of some sort.

DATA BASES

Index Medicus is available online through the MEDLARS system of the National Library of Medicine (NLM) and through Bibliographic Retrieval Services, which enhances its usefulness as a quick and timely way to locate statistical information in health sciences. Also available from NLM is the Health Planning and Administration data base, which contains citations to journals covered by *Index Medicus,* the *Hospital Literature Index,* and other sources (chapter 4).

American Statistics Index is accessible through SDC and Lockheed/DIALOG, and the NTIS data base through both of these vendors as well as Bibliographic Retrieval Services.

SELECTED BIBLIOGRAPHY OF STATISTICAL SOURCES

From among the vast number of statistical reference works available in the health care field, a few have been selected and are described here. Criteria for selection are that these works are either major compilations or are representative of a particular subject or type of data that can be accessed. It should be emphasized that the list *is* representative and by no means includes even all the major sources. However, by gaining a general idea of what is available, of the types of questions likely to be asked, and of why they are being asked in the first place, the reader will be able to deal with reference questions in the area of statistics in a logical and productive fashion.

12.1 Bureau of the Census. *Statistical Abstract of the United States.* Washington, DC, U.S. Government Printing Office, 1878– .

The *Statistical Abstract* is one of the first places to look when answering any statistical question, not just those related to health care. Published annually since 1878, this single-volume work contains more than 1,500 statistical tables and charts, which address the nation's social organization, economy, politics, and, most importantly for us, the nation's health. In the *Statistical Abstract* one can find everything from population density to the average price per pound of the catch of America's fisheries. It is, in short, an indispensable reference tool for any library.

The major strength of the *Statistical Abstract* lies in the fact that it serves as a primary and secondary source for a wide range of national statistical data. It essentially consists of excerpts, summaries, or compilations of data gathered and published in greater detail elsewhere. The original publications, both governmental and private, are always cited and can be referred to if more specificity is required.

Although the *Statistical Abstract* is published yearly, the data contained within are usually presented in multiyear groupings. There is, however, no guarantee on the currency of data or consistency of presentation from table to table, graph to graph, etc. In the 1977 edition, for example, some of the figures presented are as recent as 1977, but in some cases the most recent data may be as much as five years old. Furthermore, the data, although extensive, are not presented on a state-by-state basis. Regional subdivisions are only occasionally provided.

The basic organization of the *Statistical Abstract* has remained fairly consistent over the years: broad subject sections, appendixes, and a strong index emphasizing the subject approach. Each section, in turn, contains an explanatory preface that clearly defines major terms, concepts, and issues. As a reflection of the times, more health-related data, beginning with the 1977 edition, are being included in two sections, "Vital Statistics" and "Health and Nutrition." Additional relevant material is contained in the sections on "Population," "Social Insurance and Welfare Services," "Banking, Finance, and Insurance," "Science," and "Comparative International Statistics."

The appendixes of the *Statistical Abstract* contain, among other things, a list of "Standard Metropolitan Statistical Areas," a broad though useful guide to sources of statistics, and a list of state statistical abstracts. The most important appendix, however, is that entitled "Statistical Methodology and Reliability." Begun in 1976, this section "attempts, briefly and in nontechnical language, to provide the user a general appreciation of some of the hazards which ought to be kept in mind when putting the data to work and, in a number of specific cases, with a better understanding of how the data were collected, a measure of validity and references to further readings" (Preface).

12.2 National Center for Health Statistics. *Facts at Your Fingertips: A Guide to Sources of Statistical Information on Major Health Topics.* Hyattsville, MD, 1976– .

This *Guide* is one of the easiest to use of all statistical sources— perhaps because it does not contain any statistics! What it does have are references, names, and phone numbers, making it a good example of the general strategy outlined previously. For each topic covered, the National Center for Health Statistics has noted first which of its own publications contains relevant statistics and then has listed other organizations, both federal and private, including addresses, phone numbers, and, in some cases, the name of a contact person, making it the key to a wealth of unpublished information.

Facts at Your Fingertips is not a comprehensive source, but it is a quick first place to check and, for those areas it does cover, extremely useful. It is particularly good for locating statistics on chronic conditions such as hypoglycemia or neurological diseases, which may not be readily available elsewhere. Nor is it limited to disease information; statistical sources for adoptions, divorce, Medicare and Medicaid are some of the other topics included.

12.3 *Standard Medical Almanac.* Chicago, IL, Marquis Academic Media, 1977.

A new reference work, the *Standard Medical Almanac* states that its purpose is "to provide a comprehensive picture of the nation's health care industry," and by doing so, it vividly reflects the industry's socioeconomic and political importance. The volume consists entirely of reprints from other published sources organized into six sections: "Manpower," "Income and Expenditures," "Education and Licensure," "Facilities," "Disease and Disability," and "Federal Government and Health Care," with three indexes.

The *Almanac* is a work of exceeding volume, yet with some severe drawbacks. Most libraries, for example, will already own the original sources, but the benefits of having such a plethora of diverse information in one volume is clear. Of the three indexes, the two on organizations and geographic location are quite helpful, while the potentially valuable subject index is lacking in many respects. The original sources of the material are always given, but inasmuch as the excerpts are generally complete in and of themselves, one cannot really use the *Almanac* as a secondary source.

While it does not attempt to synthesize the data it contains, the *Standard Medical Almanac* is, in the final analysis, a good first source in answering a wide range of health-related statistical questions.

Demographic

12.4 Bureau of the Census. *Census of the Population*. Washington, DC, Bureau of the Census. Decennial.

12.5 ———. *County and City Data Book*. Washington, DC, U.S. Government Printing Office, 1949– .

12.6 ———. *Congressional District Data Book*. Washington, DC, U.S. Government Printing Office. Biennial.

12.7 ———. *Current Population Reports*. Washington, DC, U.S. Government Printing Office. Irregular.

The *Census* and its "spin-offs," listed above, provide the most thoroughly detailed data available on the population and the interaction of the population with social and economic forces. The statistics in the two "Data Books" draw not only from the *Census of the Population* but also from censuses on housing, governments, manufacturers, business, mineral industries, and agriculture, as well as updated population information. Each "Data Book" provides data broken down by the geographic divisions indicated in the title, with the *Congressional District Data Book* being the most frequently issued (one per Congress). *Current Population Reports* consists of special studies and updates irregularly issued. While there may be some question as to why these items should be included with medical and health statistics, much research today is moving in the direction of looking at the nation's health in the light of the social and economic forces that these sources reveal. Furthermore, none of the "raw data" of vital statistics can be interpreted meaningfully without reference to the population. Frequently, statistical figures are expressed in "rates," for example, the birth rate, fertility rate, or death rate. Most often this means the number of occurrences per 1,000 or per 100,000 of the population in a particular area. Accurate population statistics are thus basic to the reporting of nearly all other types of statistical information.

Vital Statistics

12.8 Bureau of the Census. *Historical Statistics of the United States; Colonial Times to 1970*. Bicentennial ed. Washington, DC, 1975.

Historical Statistics explicitly serves as a companion piece to the *Statistical Abstract:* the scope of coverage is identical, the mode of presentation is similar, and its usefulness as both a primary and secondary source endow it with equal importance. The publication pattern, however, differs, there having been only two previous editions (1949 and 1960).

Historical Statistics is organized by broad subject chapters similar, though not identical, to those of the *Statistical Abstract* and by "time series." A "time series" refers to a single vertical column of data, each increment of which extends the data backwards over time. A table of data, in turn, consists of several time series grouped together. The "Time Period Index" correlates the chapter headings with twenty-year periods in our country's history and uses the time series, rather than page numbers, as points of reference. Furthermore, an appendix in the *Statistical Abstract,* "Historical Series—Index to Tables in which Historical Statistics Appear," correlates appropriate time series in the *Historical Statistics* with the corresponding table in the current volume. By noting the time series, therefore, one can easily turn to the *Statistical Abstract* for more current data. Unfortunately, no provision was made for such ease of movement from the more recent data to the historical.

Most of the chapters are subdivided, "Migration," for example, consisting of "Internal Migration" and "International Migration and Nationalization." Each subdivision contains a preface, keyed, once again, to the various time series, which provides definitions, principles of data collection, primary sources of the data, and other important information. One cannot overlook the importance of such prefatory matter, as it obviously impinges upon possible uses of the data.

Historical Statistics is rich in information and, like the *Statistical Abstract,* is an appropriate starting point in answering any statistical question with an historical emphasis.

12.9 National Center for Health Statistics. *Vital Statistics of the United States.* Washington, DC, U.S. Government Printing Office. 1937– . Vol. 1: Natality; Vol. 2: Mortality; Vol. 3: Marriage and Divorce.

Although perpetually out of date by at least three years, *Vital Statistics of the United States* nevertheless comprises the final word on births, deaths, fetal deaths, marriages, and divorces in the United

States. The series is issued yearly, but multiyear trends are often contained in the extensive and often surprising geographic detail, occasionally down to the township level. The presence of other demographic parameters such as race, sex, and age encourages consultation of the volumes for questions that initially appear to be either too local or too particular in scope for inclusion in a "national" series. One can find, for example, such esoteric information as "Live Births by Age of Mother, Live Birth Order, and Race" for a particular state without having to locate that state's own separately published vital statistics.

The series contains no index. A highly detailed table of contents can provide adequate access if the user has already gained some familiarity with the work. In addition, volume I contains a chart, "General Pattern of Vital Registration and Statistics in the United States," which illustrates the process by which a birth, death, marriage, or divorce actually enters the reporting system. A "Technical Appendix" to each volume provides historical information, definitions, forms, and tables, which explain further the means by which people and events become statistics.

12.10 National Center for Health Statistics. *Monthly Vital Statistics Report; Provisional Statistics from the National Center for Health Statistics.* Hyattsville, MD, 1952– .

Monthly Vital Statistics Report (MVSR) is a preview of the data that will later appear in *Vital Statistics of the United States.* Each issue covers one month, providing figures on live births, deaths, natural increase in the population, marriages, divorces, and infant deaths. Multiyear trends are charted, and comparative statistics are given for the month covered in previous years as well as twelve-month cumulations. Each issue also contains state and regional statistics; age, color, and sex breakdowns on death rates; and, like the *Vital Statistics of the United States,* uses the *International Classification of Diseases* for cause of death.

The data in *MVSR* are provisional; however, the detail for which *Vital Statistics of the United States* is noted is naturally absent from the smaller publication. Most of the data in *MVSR* are based on samples rather than whole populations and are thereby subject to error.

The strengths of this newsletter, however, certainly more than compensate for its weaknesses. One can approach it for currency and constancy. Data provided are usually for the third month preceding month of issue. Since it carries the same type of information from month to month, one quickly learns what to expect from it. *Monthly Vital Statistics Report,* in short, belies its humble exterior and should find regular use in those collections where demographic information and vital statistics are in demand.

12.11   National Center for Health Statistics. *Vital and Health Statistics* series. Hyattsville, MD, 1963– .

Also known as the "Rainbow Series," the *Vital and Health Statistics* series exemplifies one of the great paradoxes of statistical reference: that data contained in it represent the National Center for Health Statistics at its best. Access to the data shows them at their worst. *Vital and Health Statistics* actually consists of thirteen irregularly issued subseries of data compiled through the surveys and studies of the NCHS. Not only are the actual data presented, but also samples of the questionnaires, technical definitions, and the like. One can find everything from "Blood Pressure Levels of Persons 6–74 Years, U.S. 1971–1974" to "Hospital and Surgical Insurance Coverage, U.S. 1974."

Or, it would be better to say, one can hope to find such data. The series's own "Current Listing and Topical Index" woefully lacks indexing appropriate to the subject matter. One cannot efficiently go to *Vital and Health Statistics* directly as a source of information. Only if a specific issue has been covered by *Index Medicus, Medical Socioeconomic Research Sources,* or has been analyzed in one's own card catalog do the efforts of those who create the series reach fruition. As is often true, *American Statistics Index* is perhaps the best key.

Nevertheless, the Rainbow Series is a must for every reference librarian. Series 10 and 11, which cover the Health Interview Survey and the Health Examination Survey, are particularly important because they contain prevalence data on chronic diseases collected by NCHS and unavailable elsewhere on a national scale. The various subseries and the areas they cover are listed below.

VITAL AND HEALTH STATISTICS SERIES[9]

Series 1.   *Programs and Collection Procedures.* Reports that describe the general programs of the National Center for Health Statistics and its offices and divisions and data collection methods used and include definitions and other material necessary for understanding the data

Series 2. *Data Evaluation and Methods Research.* Studies of new statistical methodology, including experimental tests of new survey methods, studies of vital statistics collection methods, new analytical techniques, objective evaluations of reliability of collected data, and contributions to statistical theory

Series 3. *Analytical Studies.* Reports presenting analytical or interpretive studies based on vital and health statistics, carrying the analysis further than the expository types of reports in the other series

Series 4. *Documents and Committee Reports.* Final reports of major committees concerned with vital and health statistics and documents such as recommended model vital registration laws and revised birth and death certificates

Series 10. *Data From the Health Interview Survey.* Statistics on illness, accidental injuries, disability, use of hospital, medical, dental, and other services, and other health-related topics, all based on data collected in a continuing national household interview survey

Series 11. *Data From the Health Examination Survey and the Health and Nutrition Examination Survey.* Data from direct examination, testing, and measurement of national samples of the civilian noninstitutionalized population provide the basis for two types of reports: (1) estimates of the medically defined prevalence of specific disease in the United States and the distribution of the population with respect to physical, physiological, and psychological characteristics and (2) analysis of relationships among the various measurements without reference to an explicit finite universe of persons

Series 12. *Data From the Institutionalized Population Surveys.* Discontinued effective 1975. Future reports from these surveys will be in Series 13

Series 13. *Data on Health Resources Utilization.* Statistics on the utilization of health manpower and facilities providing long-term care, ambulatory care, hospital care, and family planning services

Series 14. *Data on Health Resources: Manpower and Facilities.* Statistics on the numbers, geographic distribution, and characteristics of health resources, including physicians, dentists, nurses, other health occupations, hospitals, nursing homes, and outpatient facilities

Series 20. *Data on Mortality.* Various statistics on mortality other than as included in regular annual or monthly reports. Special analysis by cause of death, age, and other demographic variables; geographic and time series analyses; and statistics on characteristics of death not available from the vital records based on sample surveys of those records

Series 21. *Data on Natality, Marriage, and Divorce.* Various statistics on natality, marriage, and divorce other than as included in regular annual or monthly reports. Special analyses by demographic variables; geographic and time series analyses; studies of fertility; and statistics on characteristics of birth not available from the vital records based on sample surveys of those records

Series 22. *Data From the National Mortality and Natality Surveys.* Discontinued effective 1975. Future reports from these sample surveys based on vital records will be included in Series 20 and 21, respectively

Series 23. *Data From the National Survey of Family Growth.* Statistics on fertility, family formation and dissolution, family planning, and related maternal and infant health topics derived from a biennial survey of a nationwide probability sample of ever-married women 15–44 years of age.

12.12 National Center for Health Statistics. *Advance Data from Vital and Health Statistics of the National Center for Health Statistics.* Hyattsville, MD, 1976– .

The full title to *Advance Data,* provided in the above citation, accurately describes this short (5–10 pages), irregularly issued newsletter: a vehicle by which information from the various surveys conducted by the National Center for Health Statistics gains early release to the public. Most of the information contained in *Advance Data* will eventually find its way into the *Vital and Health Statistics* series. Each issue addresses only one topic, ranging from "Wanted and Unwanted Births Reported by Mothers 15–44 years of Age: United States, 1973" to "Height and Weight of Adults 18–74 Years of Age in the United States," and is replete with the necessary charts and tables, footnotes, cross-references, definitions, forms, and technical notes.

Advance Data, however, suffers acutely from the weakness of the other government-issued statistical series: the wealth of information remains a hidden treasure due to lack of subject access. The publication has no index itself, and *American Statistics Index* stands alone among the major tools that provide coverage. Nor does there seem to be any pattern of topics that could reliably provide direction to its contents. *Advance Data*, in short, must be monitored to be utilized effectively.

12.13 Center for Disease Control. *MMWR: Morbidity and Mortality Weekly Report*. Atlanta, GA, 1952– .

At the heart of *MMWR* are four statistical tables: I. Cases of specified notifiable diseases, United States (for week covered and cumulative for the year); II. Notifiable diseases of low frequency, United States (cumulative for the year only); III. Cases of specified notifiable diseases, United States (for week covered only and that week of the preceding year, by geographic region); and IV. Deaths in 121 United States cities (for one week only). These tables provide the user with extremely current data on the occurrence of various diseases in the country.

Each issue also contains three to five special sections: "Surveillance Summary," "Epidemiologic Notes and Reports," "Current Trends," "Recommendation of the Public Health Service Advisory Committee on Immunization Practice," and "International Notes." These, and the topics they address, vary from week to week, but they provide larger pictures on items of interest both nationally and internationally. A "Surveillance Summary," for example, might cover rabies in the United States for a single year. A specific outbreak of legionnaires' disease would be reported in "Epidemiologic Notes and Reports."

An annual supplement augments *MMWR*, summarizing the weekly statistical data and containing, among other things, a list of state epidemiologists. The supplement does not, however, supersede the special reports in the weekly issues, which should be retained. Nor does the supplement provide an index to the valuable and interesting information contained in the articles, the *American Statistics Index* being the only major tool that does so. In providing morbidity data, *MMWR* complements *Monthly Vital Statistics Report* in providing current information on the nation's health.

12.14 Center for Disease Control. *Surveillance Reports*. Atlanta, GA. Multiple series. Irregular.

The *Surveillance Reports* consist of numerous summaries of data received from around the nation on various conditions. Congenital malformations, trichinosis, malaria, hepatitis, and abortion are but five of the more than twenty topics covered. The titles, conditions surveyed, and frequency of issue vary. Bibliographic control is spotty at best—these are not depository items—so close monitoring and regular communication with the CDC is necessary to establish and maintain current information on a host of communicable diseases, preventable conditions, or any other health topic the CDC has decided to oversee.

12.15 National Cancer Institute. *Cancer Patient Survival*. Report No. 5– , 1977– .

An example of a very comprehensive and specialized type of statistical publication, *Cancer Patient Survival* is published by the National Cancer Institute and contains sampling data from reporting hospitals in the United States. Reports 1–4 were titled *End Results in Cancer—Cancer Patient Survival,* giving perhaps a more optimistic touch to the data. Several different survival measures are shown for thirty-nine different types of cancer. Data are presented separately for blacks and whites.

12.16 National Center for Health Statistics. *Selected National Data Sources for Health Planners*. Hyattsville, MD, 1976.

Selected National Data Sources for Health Planners is a secondary source compiled by the National Center for Health Statistics. It contains references to the "most useful sources of data" for state and local health planners. One of the mandates of Public Law 93–641, the National Health Planning and Resources Development Act of 1974, is that Health Systems Agencies must utilize *existing* data in their activities as much as possible—in other words, a request not to redescribe the statistical wheel.

Whether you are a health sciences reference librarian in a large university with a school of public health, in a Health Systems Agency library, or in a small hospital library, you will find such data more and more in demand. If new to the field of statistical reference work, you will find this source a good overview of everything that is available from national sources in the area of health statistics. Section A briefly discusses the Cooperative Health Statistics System and what is being done by various government agencies in the collection of statistics.

The remainder of the work lists sources of information in all the usual areas—health care resources (facilities and utilization), national health care programs, health economics (expenditures), and sources of demographic data. Both printed sources and data available on magnetic tape are included. For each source, the name of the federal agency (with a contact address) is given, along with coverage characteristics of the data, such as time period, geographic area, exactly what information is included, and date of next revision.

12.17 National Center for Health Services Research. *Health: United States.* Washington, DC, U.S. Government Printing Office.

Health: United States consists of reports to the Congress required by the Public Health Services Act. How much is spent in the United States for health care, where this money comes from, and how it is allocated are addressed in the first section. The remaining information summarizes statistics on a wide variety of topics relating to health manpower, facilities, and the health status of the population. More detailed information on all of these subjects can be found elsewhere, and *Health: United States* indicates this in footnotes throughout.

12.18 National Center for Health Statistics. *Health Resources Statistics.* Washington, DC, U.S. Government Printing Office, 1965– .

Health Resources Statistics is a summary of data regarding health manpower, facilities, and services compiled by the Division of Health Manpower and Facilities Statistics of the National Center for Health Statistics. It "is intended to provide current and comprehensive statistics on a wide range of health areas as baseline data for the planning, administration and evaluation of health programs" (Summary, p. vii). Most of this information was not in fact generated by the National Center for Health Statistics, however, but was compiled and interpreted by them from the "best available sources." These sources—whether published or not—are identified at the end of each chapter and may be consulted for further information. *Health Resources Statistics* has an index, appendixes on certification and licensure, and introductory chapters that discuss the nature and reliability of the statistical information it contains.

A few examples of the types of questions that can be answered from *Health Resources Statistics* are the following: "What institutions offer training in the various health professions?" "How many persons are employed in each of these professions?" "What are their job titles?" "Where are such health facilities as blood banks, poison control centers, and family planning services located, and how many are there?"

A problem with *Health Resources Statistics*—as with all such compilations—is the currency of the data. Most is at least several years old and, where more current information is sought, the only solution is to contact the appropriate agency, if it can be found, or NCHS itself.

12.19 American Hospital Association. *Hospital Statistics.* Chicago, IL, 1972– .

Help for statistical questions about health facilities may be found in Series 13 of the *Vital and Health Statistics* series—*Data on Health Resources Utilization.* A more up-to-date source for hospitals themselves is *Hospital Statistics,* containing information garnered by the American Hospital Association in its annual survey of hospitals. A short introduction defines terms used and discusses trends in hospital utilization and characteristics. Following are tables containing the previous year's data on utilization, personnel, finances, facilities, services, and special beds broken down by census divisions and by state. *Hospital Statistics* is the place to go for answers to such questions as "What percentage of hospitals in Mississippi have speech pathology services?" or "How many hospital beds are there in the state of Maryland?"

Another source of information on hospitals is *Length of Stay in PAS (Professional Activity Study) Hospitals, by Diagnosis,* compiled by the Commission on Professional and Hospital Activities. As the Preface notes, "These statistics can provide a valuable perspective for physicians, administrators, PSROs (Professional Standards Review Organizations), and planners who make decisions based on length of hospitalization." It can also help answer such questions as "Is there a difference in average length of hospital stay for bone cancer between patients over 65 and those under 20?"

12.20 American Medical Association. *Physician Distribution and Medical Licensure in the U.S.* Chicago, IL 1975– .

Formerly known as the "Distribution of Physicians" series, *Physician Distribution and Medical Licensure* is the *sine qua non* of physician manpower statistics. Not only is it the best location for information on how many doctors work where, but its already considerable virtue has been greatly enhanced by the addition of the "Annual Report of Medical Licensure Statistics," previously published in the *Journal of the American Medical Association*. Extensive tables provide information on the number of physicians by major professional activity for nation, region, state, metropolitan area, and county. Hospital and population data are given together for comparative purposes, as well as per capita income for the geographic region covered. At the state level a breakdown by physician specialty is given. Although many socioeconomic data of interest, such as physician income, hours worked per week, and minority and female representation, are not included here, *Physician Distribution* is still an indispensable reference tool.

12.21 American Medical Association. *Reference Data on Profile of Medical Practice*. Chicago, IL, 1971– .

12.22 ———. *Reference Data on Socioeconomic Issues of Health*. Chicago, IL, 1971– .

Taken together, the Red Book and the Blue Book, as they are respectively known, give the American Medical Association's picture of health care in the United States. The *Profile of Medical Practice* contains information on physicians—their numbers, income, expenses, specialties, and practice characteristics, gathered by the AMA itself. *Socioeconomic Issues of Health* is a quick reference guide to data that can be found more comprehensively in other sources; some of these have been mentioned here. Summary information on, to name just a few topics, health insurance, hospital utilization, and population characteristics is included. Both these books are small enough so that the librarian can become familiar with the data they contain, which is fortunate, since only the briefest of indexes is included.

International

12.23 World Health Organization. *World Health Statistics Quarterly*. Geneva, 1978– . (Continues *Epidemiological and Vital Statistics Report*, 1947–67; *World Health Statistics Report*, 1968–77.)

12.24 ———. *World Health Statistics Annual*. Geneva, 1939– .

Both are published by the World Health Organization (WHO) and attempt to give a picture of health and vital statistics on a worldwide basis. A cautionary note: the statistical expressions are only as good as the reporting system in each country, and these vary widely in consistency and reliability. Giving some recognition to this problem,

WHO has set up an information service on world health statistics, which, among other things, aims to improve the quality and timeliness of information available and to define the limiting factors caused by comparing data generated from many different sources.

World Health Statistics Annual contains final and "official" (i.e., given to WHO by the "competent authorities" of the countries concerned) vital statistics, morbidity statistics for infectious diseases, and information on health resources, usually published several years after the fact. For example, volumes published in 1978 contain data relevant "mainly to 1975 and 1976." The *Annual* continues a tradition of reporting this information first begun by the League of Nations with its *Annual Epidemiological Report* for 1921–38 and then taken up by WHO in the *Annual Epidemiological and Vital Statistics* for 1939–46.

The *Annual* is published in three parts. Volume I contains vital statistics—including population, natality, mortality, and infant mortality—breaking down mortality further by causes of death selected from the "A List" of the *International Classification of Diseases.* Information includes total numbers and rates, proportions of deaths by sex and causes at all ages, and numbers and rates also by age.

Volume II presents data on reported cases of infectious diseases and deaths from infectious diseases. Arrangement again follows the *International Classification of Diseases.* Volume III gives information on worldwide health personnel and hospital establishments, including both actual numbers and ratios for selected occupations. Data on hospitals include number of beds, admissions, discharges, and utilization measures. Like many statistical publications, the *World Health Statistics Annual* contains a great deal of useful information hidden between its covers. There is no index—the only solution seems to be familiarity with the publication and the types of questions it will be able to answer.

World Health Statistics Quarterly (formerly *World Health Statistics Report*) is, as the title implies, an ongoing, more frequently published medium for providing data on various aspects of world health statistics. What is reported varies with each issue. There are two sections—one on "Special Subjects," for example, sex differentials in mortality in Arab countries. The other section is "Current Data"—always including data on some infectious diseases and on hospitals, health personnel, or vital statistics. The *Quarterly* is indexed in *Index Medicus.*

12.25 United Nations. *Demographic Yearbook.* Statistical Office, New York, NY, 1948– .

Published by the United Nations, the *Yearbook* is the official source of international demographic statistics. As such, it supplements the *World Health Statistics Quarterly* and the *World Health Statistics Annual* with more detailed demographic information than they contain. It also offers (in the "Technical Notes" preceding the tables) a detailed explanation of the variables included, the reliability of the present data, and the earlier data with which they can be compared.

REFERENCES

[1] U.S. Congress. House. Committee on Interstate and Foreign Commerce, Subcommittee on Health and the Environment. *A Discursive Dictionary of Health Care.* Washington, DC, United States Government Printing Office, 1976.

[2] National Center for Health Statistics. *Policy Statement.* Washington, DC, United States Government Printing Office, 1978. p. 1.

[3] "History of Collection in the United States Vital Statistics System." *Vital Statistics of the United States,* Washington, DC, United States Government Printing Office, Vol. I, 1950. p. 2–19.

[4] All publications listed here, as well as other major compilations of statistical data, are described in more detail at the end of this chapter.

[5] *1977/78 United States Government Manual.* Washington, DC, United States Government Printing Office, 1978. p. 262.

[6] U.S. Congress. House. *op. cit.,* p. 26.

[7] National Library of Medicine. *Medical Subject Headings, Annotated Alphabetic List, 1979.* Springfield, VA, NTIS, 1978. p. LV–LXI.

[8] *American Statistics Index, 4th Annual Supplement.* Washington, DC, Congressional Information Service, 1978, Index. p. vii.

[9] National Center for Health Statistics. *Mailing List Request Form.* HRA-T60 (7/77). Hyattsville, MD, 1977.

CHAPTER 13

Directories
and
Biographical Sources

JO ANNE BOORKMAN

Directories are among the most frequently consulted reference tools, and one of the major factors to consider when dealing with them is currency. The *Federal Executive Telephone Directory*, for example, is updated every two months to reflect the continuous changes in government. This is probably an extreme example; nevertheless, the accuracy of the information a librarian is able to provide will be related to the timeliness of the directories in the collection.

Another factor to consider in selecting and using directories is their format. Often, in a reference situation, the patron is in a hurry, and the librarian needs to locate the answer as quickly as possible. It can, therefore, be frustrating to have to flip through a directory, hoping to find the needed section, or to hunt for an index buried in the middle of the volume. Some directories conveniently have an alphabetical arrangement. Others frequently are arranged geographically or in a classified subject format. Without an index, these can be tedious to use, especially if the requester does not have sufficient information to be helpful. It is imperative that the librarian know his or her directories.

BIOGRAPHICAL SOURCES AND
DIRECTORIES OF SCIENTISTS

Some of the most frequent reference requests are for biographical or address information. A patron wants to know the educational background of a physician before making an appointment, or an insurance company needs to confirm the address of a physician. These questions often appear to be very straightforward and uncomplicated. However, the patron does not always know the first name of Dr. Smith in Los Angeles, and Dr. Smith's specialty may be internal medicine, but then again it may be gastroenterology. The insurance secretary just has the doctor's signature, and it "looks like" T. J. Crandell, or is that F. J. Granville? Thus, two seemingly direct requests for information are often less than clear. With biographical questions it is important to find out as much information from the patron as possible. Some questions to consider:

Is the person living or dead?
What field of medicine or science does the person work in?
Does the person work with a university or research institution, or in a hospital?
Has the person published any books or journal articles?
What country does the person live in?

Often the only information about a person is a listing in a society roster or an address in a journal article. This is especially true for people who are just establishing themselves in a field.

The biographical sources and directories discussed in this chapter are examples of major sources. There are innumerable directories of professional societies, and the most obvious and frequently over- looked source is the telephone directory. These will not be discussed here. The following sources are primarily for physicians and scientists in the United States, with a few examples of directories to scientists in Great Britain and other countries.

United States

13.1 *American Men and Women of Science*. 14th ed. New York, NY, Cattell/Bowker, 1979. 8 vols.

13.2 *American Men and Women of Science: The Medical and Health Sciences, 1977*. New York, NY, Cattell/Bowker, 1977.

Now in its fourteenth edition, *American Men and Women of Science (AMWS)* provides biographical sketches of scientists from the United States and Canada in an alphabetical arrangement. Selection for in- clusion is based on (1) achievement by experience or stature derived from doctoral or current research, (2) published scientific research (or the judgment of peers for classified research), (3) attainment of a position of substantial responsibility requiring a scientific background equivalent to criteria 1 and 2. The directory provides brief biographical information, professional experience, present position, professional memberships, and major publications. Inclusion in the directory is by nomination and evaluation by other scientists, based on the individual's research and publications. A special feature of this directory is a necrology section at the end of each volume.

The *American Men and Women of Science: The Medical and Health Sciences* is a subset of the thirteenth edition of *AMWS* and includes 26,500 entries. Entries are the same as those in *AMWS* with the same criteria for inclusion. To keep the directory compact, some of the information is abbreviated, with a list of abbreviations in the front of the volume. This would be a good directory for smaller libraries that might find it difficult to justify purchasing the *American Men and Women of Science*.

13.3 *American Medical Directory.* 21st ed. Chicago, IL, American Medical Association, 1979. 4 pts.

The twenty-first edition of *American Medical Directory* was published in early 1979. The *Directory* formerly was published every two years as a directory of all physicians in the United States and its territories and possessions, with AMA members indicated in boldface type. The first part of the directory is an alphabetical listing of physicians, giving their city and state of residence. The other three parts make up a geographical register by state and city, which provides coded information about each physician: address, year of birth, medical school and year of degree, year of licensure, year of national board certification, specialty board(s), society membership, and type of practice. Full listings deciphering the codes are in a special section.

13.4 *Directory of Medical Specialists.* Chicago, IL, Marquis. Vol. 1– , 1939– . Annual.

This directory, which now appears in two volumes each year, lists physicians certified by recognized medical specialty boards sponsored by national societies and the corresponding scientific sections of the AMA. Each board is listed separately with a brief historical sketch, a description of the board's purpose, certification information, and the board's address. A register of members by state and city follows. A brief biographical sketch, based on information solicited by questionnaire, contains many abbreviations; in addition to information on medical school, internship, residency, and postdoctoral education, the individual's clinical training and professional membership(s) are listed. A name index in the back of volume 2 lists the physician's city, state, and specialty. A physician certified by more than one board will be listed for each, but biographical information will be listed only under one specialty. This directory is frequently useful when a patron wants to know how "good" a physician is. It may be reassuring for a patron to see which physicians are certified and to read about their education and professional training.

This directory, besides giving more information for each physician, is published more frequently than the *American Medical Directory* and is therefore more current in its information. The currency of a directory is often of major importance; when giving a patron directory information, it is a good idea to note source and date. The information contained, as well as the physicians listed, is only as complete as the questionnaires that were submitted.

The remaining items in this section are examples of directories published by professional organizations. All require certain minimum qualifications for membership.

13.5   American College of Surgeons. *Yearbook*. Chicago, IL, 1953– . Annual.

13.6   American College of Hospital Administrators. *Directory: a comprehensive biographical directory of the entire membership, including an ACHA district index*. Chicago, IL, 1960– . Biennial.

13.7   *American Dental Directory*. Chicago, IL, American Dental Association, 1947– . Annual.

13.8   American Veterinary Medical Association. *Directory*. Chicago, IL, 1978. Biennial, even-numbered years.

13.9   Federation of American Societies for Experimental Biology. *Directory of Members*. Bethesda, MD, 1964/65– . Annual.

13.10   *Who's Who in Health Care*. New York, NY, Hanover Publications, Inc., 1977.

The *Yearbook* of the American College of Surgeons provides brief biographical sketches of members, including hospital affiliations and titles. Some foreign physicians are listed. Members are not necessarily certified by the American Board of Surgery, but all must meet the requirements of the College to be listed as fellows.

The *Directory* of the American College of Hospital Administrators uses a format similar to that of the *Directory of Medical Specialists* and gives a complete professional biography. Member requirements are explicit: nominees must have either a Bachelor of Arts degree with three years of hospital administration experience or a Master of Science degree and one year's experience. Nominees are accepted for membership after having passed both oral and written examinations. Both nominees and full members are included in the directory.

The *American Dental Directory*, like its medical counterpart, tries to list all dentists, not just American Dental Association members. The coded information provides a professional biography for each dentist, including information on dental education, year of graduation, and type of practice. Also included in the directory are a number of other listings: a list of dental schools; state, national, and world dental organizations; and the number of dentists in various countries.

In similar format, the *Directory* of the American Veterinary Association tries to provide professional biographical sketches of all veterinarians, not just its members.

The Federation of American Societies for Experimental Biology is an association of six member societies (the American Physiological Society, the American Society of Biological Chemists, the American Society for Pharmacology and Experimental Therapeutics, the American Institute for Nutrition, the American Society for Experimental Pathology, and the American Association of Immunologists), and their *Directory of Members* provides a consolidated alphabetical listing of all members with addresses and phone numbers. There is also a geographical list of members, as well as organizational information— officers, committees, and constitution—for each society.

Who's Who in Health Care was published to bring together in one source biographical information about leaders in all aspects of health care. Altogether, 8,000 biographies are presented in an alphabetical arrangement. Inclusion in this directory, as with the others mentioned, follows certain criteria based either on one's position of responsibility or one's meritorious contribution to health care as judged by the editorial advisory board. A geographic index and a classified index (occupations, health facilities, organizations, government, private industry, etc.) complete the volume. Individuals from the United States and Canada represent the majority of the listings, although a few representatives from other countries are also present.

Great Britain

Information about British scientists and physicians is frequently requested.

These two directories cover scientists in all fields, but are somewhat dated:

13.11   *Directory of British Scientists.* 3d ed. London, Binn, 1966.

13.12   *Who's Who of British Scientists.* 1969/70–1971/72. London, Longmans, 1970.

The Directory of British Scientists, covering 54,000 scientists, is the British equivalent of the *American Men and Women of Science.* "Pure science" is emphasized, and entries are given in a classified arrangement by discipline, with an alphabetical name index. Biographical information includes name, address, phone number, current position, degrees obtained, and important writings. The directory also lists scientific societies, their journals and editors, and government and private research institutions.

Who's Who of British Scientists lists 10,000 men and women in the biological sciences—again, in a classified arrangement by discipline.

The two directories of British physicians are both published annually; both also include physicians outside Great Britain and are useful for locating physicians residing in Commonwealth countries.

13.13   *Medical Directory.* London, Churchill. Annual.

13.14   *Medical Register.* London, General Medical Council. Annual.

The *Medical Directory,* a commercial publication, lists physicians registered with the General Medical Council. The alphabetically arranged biographies include address, education, and some publications, for physicians primarily in England, Scotland, Wales, and Ireland. There is a geographical index as well as lists of universities, colleges, medical schools, hospitals, medical offices of health, government departments, coroners, medical societies, and medical periodicals.

The *Medical Register* is the official listing of physicians, and "inclusion in this list constitutes for physicians a legal right to practice." The alphabetical listing gives a physician's name, address, registration date, and degrees, and includes foreign medical graduates certified to practice medicine in Great Britain. The *Register* is useful for locating practitioners in the Commonwealth, especially Australia and

New Zealand, albeit limited to those licensed in the United Kingdom. The *Medical Register* also provides information for certification.

Other Countries

Many other countries publish directories of physicians and other health personnel and institutions.

> 13.15 *Canadian Medical Directory.* Don Mills, Ont., Seccombe House. Annual.
> 13.16 *Guide Rosenwald Médical et Pharmaceutical.* Paris, Expansion Scientifique Française. Annual.

These two directories, both commercially published, provide lists of physicians both alphabetically and geographically, although their formats are otherwise different. The Canadian directory provides brief biographical information alphabetically for each physician who returned a questionnaire, including year and school of medical degree, professional memberships, position and hospital affiliation(s), address, and telephone number. Abbreviations used in this section are listed in the front of the directory. The geographical listing gives only the physician's name and specialty under province and city. A third section of the directory lists universities, societies, governmental departments, and officials, as well as miscellaneous items ranging from venereal disease regulations and poison control centers to statistics on distances and areas. Official lists of Canadian physicians are published annually by the provincial licensing authorities and are available through the Provincial Colleges of Physicians and Surgeons.

The *Guide Rosenwald* has a rainbow of sections listing physicians, pharmacists, hospitals, public assistance establishments, medical laboratories, and "stations hydro-climatiques" (the latter includes the curative nature of the waters at each). This directory also contains advertising throughout.

International

Some of the people most difficult to locate are those outside of the English-speaking countries. In addition to *Guide Rosenwald*, the following directories help; however, since they are selective, only the well-known, deceased, or older scientists will be included. The directories do serve very well in providing brief biographical information for those individuals they cover.

13.17   *Who's Who in Science in Europe: A Reference Guide to European Scientists.* 3d ed. Guernsey, Channel Islands, G. Hodgson, 1978. 4 vols.

13.18   Turkevich, J., and Turkevich, L. B. *Prominent Scientists of Continental Europe.* New York, NY, American Elsevier, 1968.

13.19   *World Who's Who in Science.* Chicago, IL, Marquis, 1968.

The first directory includes nearly 50,000 scientists from both Eastern and Western Europe in the fields of natural, physical, medical, and agricultural sciences. Information obtained from questionnaires provides birth dates and professional society memberships. No publications are listed. *Prominent Scientists of Continental Europe* also includes individuals from Eastern and Western Europe. It is very selective, however, and is limited to members of national academies and professors at leading universities. Entries are arranged alphabetically under the country of residence and include short professional biographies similar to those in *Who's Who in Science in Europe,* with the additional mention of major publications.

World Who's Who in Science lists 30,000 biographical sketches of scientists from antiquity to the present and is international in scope. Entries include personal and professional information on scientific contributions and interests. The inside front and back covers provide a list of Nobel Prize winners up to 1968.

13.20   *Current Bibliographic Directory of the Arts and Sciences.* Philadelphia, PA, Institute for Scientific Information, 1978– . Annual. (Called *International Directory of Research and Development Scientists,* 1968–70; *ISI's Who is Publishing in Science,* 1971–78.)

This, the most current international directory, is an outgrowth of *Current Contents* for the year,* providing individual author and institutional addresses. In addition, listings are included from the *Index to Science and Technology Proceedings* and in future editions will also include the *Index to Social Sciences and Humanities Proceedings.* This is an excellent source for locating little-known scientists, who have nevertheless published. With this latest edition individuals from the arts and humanities have also been included from *Current Contents, Arts and Humanities.* The author section provides the address of the first author of a paper, which is taken from the reprint address accom-

---

*Previous editions contained listings from authors who had published in the previous year.

panying a journal article, as well as abbreviated citations for books and journal articles published. The organization section of the directory is an alphabetical listing, international in scope, of over 46,000 government, academic, industrial, and other organizations; a geographical section lists the United States by state, then other countries, with the author and organization names listed below.

DIRECTORIES OF ORGANIZATIONS

Next in frequency to requests for information about people come questions about organizations. Again, addresses and telephone numbers are most often needed, although information about an organization's structure, purpose, meetings, and membership make up a great number of requests. It is important to note, even for a recent edition, how a directory obtains updated information. Directories that rely on questionnaires, for example, may have old information if a listed organization fails to send in updated information.

13.21 *Encyclopedia of Associations.* 13th ed. Detroit, MI, Gale Research Co. 3 vols. (Vol. 3 is a looseleaf supplement entitled: *Encyclopedia of Associations; New Associations and Projects.*)

13.22 *Foundation Directory.* 7th ed. New York, NY, Columbia University Press, 1979. Biennial.

13.23 *Research Centers Directory: A Guide to University-Related and Other Nonprofit Organizations.* 6th ed. Detroit, MI, Gale Research Co., 1979. (Looseleaf supplement entitled: *New Research Centers.*)

13.24 Kruzas, A. T., and Fitch, A. R., eds. *Medical and Health Information Directory.* Detroit, MI, Gale Research Co., 1977.

13.25 Norback, C. T., and Norback, P. G., eds. *The Health Care Directory.* Oradell, NJ, Medical Economics, 1977–78.

For an all-purpose directory of organizations in the United States, the *Encyclopedia of Associations* is excellent. Its scope is limited to nonprofit national organizations; that is, the parent organization of the American Cancer Society is listed, but not local, state, and regional branches or affiliates. The more than 15,000 entries are in a classified arrangement—science and technology, social welfare, education, etc. In addition to the address, telephone number, and chief officers of an organization, entries include membership size, purpose of the organization, meetings/conventions, and publications. The organizational name index provides listings by significant words in the name and supplements the name with a subject if the name is not clear. For example, the American Celiac Society is found in the index under:

American Celiac Society
Celiac Society: American
(Nutrition) American Celiac Society

The second volume provides geographic and executive indexes to the organizations, while the third volume is a supplement providing quarterly listings to new associations and projects not in the main listing.

The *Foundation Directory* features nonprofit, nongovernment organizations that have private financial backing. This directory is especially useful for individuals seeking funds for research and education. Entries are arranged geographically by state and include the address, date of establishment, donors, trustees, and purpose of the foundation, as well as its fields of interest and financial assets. Also included is grant application information. Two indexes provide access by subject and by names of persons associated with the foundations (donors, trustees, and administrators).

The *Research Centers Directory* again presents information on nonprofit research organizations; however, the directory is limited to those centers that are university sponsored. Entries are arranged by subject and include the size of the staff and monies spent on research in addition to the address and purpose of the center. Two indexes, an alphabetical index by the center's name and an institutional index of sponsoring universities, complete the main volume. A looseleaf supplement provides updated information periodically.

Kruzas' *Medical and Health Information Directory* and Norback's *Health Care Directory* both bring a great deal of information together into single volumes. The subtitle to Kruzas' work summarizes its contents:

A guide to state, national and international organizations, government agencies, educational institutions, hospitals, grant-award sources, health care delivery agencies, journals, newsletters, review

serials, abstracting services, publishers, research centers, computerized date banks, audiovisual services and libraries and information centers.

Primary access to all this information is through the table of contents. Some of the sections, e.g., "Federal Grants and Domestic Assistance" and "Audiovisual Producers," have their own indexes at
the end of their respective sections. The formats of the sections vary
with the nature of the information within. Entries in the "Research
Centers and Institutes" section look exactly like the entries in *Research
Centers Directory*, and that directory is listed in the introduction as a
source of additional information. The introduction also lists sources
for additional information related to each chapter.

This *Directory* brings together much useful information into one
compact volume, although access to the information is awkward because the indexes are buried in the body of the book. Before an
organization can be looked up, the table of contents must first be
scanned and the appropriate index located. Some sections are arranged geographically by state and then alphabetically; others are
arranged alphabetically by organization. Unfortunately, the appropriate section may not always be evident from the name of the organization or the information a patron may have. For example, a request
for the address of Health Services, Inc., would be difficult to locate
unless the patron or the librarian knew that it was a Blue Cross-Blue
Shield Plan. Likewise, a request for information on the Cardiovascular
Health Center in New York might be difficult to locate unless the
librarian happened to find it listed in the back of the book in the
Research Centers and Institutes Index. A general index to the entire
volume would make this directory more valuable as a reference tool.

The *Health Care Directory* has similar advantages and disadvantages. It provides information on health-related topics from adoption
to sex change clinics. Directories to diverse manufacturers, consultants, specialized hospitals, group practices, and audiovisual software
producers are a few of the many (and otherwise difficult to locate)
sources in the volume. Sections vary in format: manufacturer sections
like "Laboratory Equipment and Supplies" are arranged in two
parts—an alphabetical listing of manufacturers with addresses, followed by a product index (another buried index) arranged by product
name with an alphabetical list of manufacturers' names under each
product. No page numbers are given to the manufacturers' section.

Other sections, like "Group Practices," are arranged geographically by state, but if the state in which an organization is located is not known, this directory is difficult to use. Another difficulty comes from having the names of the states printed in the same type as the listings. Again, a general index would make this *Directory* even more useful.

These two directories, even with the drawbacks in their formats, are good choices for smaller libraries. They bring together a vast amount of information that could otherwise be available only with a large collection of different directories.

13.26 *Scientific, Technical and Related Societies of the United States.* 9th ed. Washington, DC, National Academy of Sciences, National Research Council, 1971.

13.27 *World Guide to Scientific Associations and Learned Scientists.* 2d ed. New York, NY, Bowker, 1978.

13.28 *Yearbook of International Organizations.* Brussels, Union of International Associations, 1948– . Irregular.

Scientific and Technical Societies in the United States, while providing more complete information about each organization than the *Encyclopedia of Associations,* is dated (9th edition, 1971). This lack of currency is a drawback in a directory that purports to provide address, officers, purpose, history, meetings, professional activities, publications, and awards that each association sponsors. Trade associations are not included.

The *World Guide to Scientific Associations and Learned Societies* is an international directory to associations and societies representing all fields of science and the arts. The body of the *World Guide* is arranged geographically by continent, then by country, with an alphabetical arrangement of entries under the country. The directory is in German and English; and each entry includes the name of the association or society, an abbreviated name, the year of the organization's founding, address, president's or director's name, and number of members. A list of subjects follows the main section of the directory. Page numbers in this list refer to the beginning of the subject listings in the index, arranged geographically under each subject by continent, country, and then organization names; but no page numbers are given referring back to the main directory, making the index tedious to use. There is, too, no name index by each organization's name; nor is there a listing of organizations alphabetically under subject. The international scope of the *World Guide* is its primary strength.

The *Yearbook of International Organizations* is not limited to science and the arts. It does, however, have definite criteria for inclusion as an "international" organization: essentially an organization must have a minimum of three countries participating in its founding, aims, structure, membership, officers, congresses, and financial backing. The organization must also have a permanent address. The directory is divided into two sections. Section A lists those organizations fulfilling the "international" criteria. Besides name and address, each listing contains information on the seven criteria mentioned above and information on publications of the organization. Section B lists those organizations that have been inactive for five years and that may be "international," but for which insufficient information was available at the time of printing. Listings here give primarily names, addresses, and chief officers of organizations. There are several indexes: name and classified indexes are in English and French, and there is also a geographical index. The indexes refer to both sections of the main directory. There is also an acronym and abbreviation listing at the end of the volume.

The *Yearbook of International Organizations* provides more information about each organization it lists, as well as more complete and easier-to-use indexes than the *World Guide*. The *World Guide*, however, is not limited to organizations "international in scope and purpose." Both are useful in locating information on organizations outside the United States.

13.29   *The AHA Guide to the Health Care Field.* Chicago, IL, American Hospital Association, 1972– . Annual (continues the Guide issue of *Hospitals*).

13.30   *Canadian Hospital Directory.* Ottawa, Ont., Canadian Hospital Association. Vol. 1– , 1953– .

The *AHA Guide* is one of the most useful directories available. It lists United States hospitals geographically by state, city, then alphabetically by hospital. Government hospitals outside the United States are also included. Each listing, in addition to the address, telephone number, and chief administrator, provides coded information on the hospital's facilities, service, governing structure, and size of staff. Accreditation by the Joint Commission on Accreditation of Hospitals (JCAH) and membership in the American Hospital Association are indicated. Brief statistical information on inpatient data (beds, admissions, census, percent occupancy), newborn data (bassinets, births), and expenses (total, payroll) are also provided. A second section lists American Hospital Association membership, including offices, officers, historical data, institutional, personal members, and associate members. The third section of the directory lists other health organizations, agencies, and universities and schools offering educational programs in health fields. A hospital buyers' guide completes the directory. The *Guide* can be tedious to use because of its geographical approach to the hospitals; however, its compact presentation makes it a valuable reference source for hospital information. A list of abbreviations used in the *Guide* and an index to manufacturers in the Buyers Guide are at the end of the volume.

The *Canadian Hospital Directory* presents similar information for Canadian hospitals. Its geographical format is in eleven sections for the ten provinces (arranged west to east) plus the Yukon and Northwest territories. Maps accompany each section, identifying towns that have hospitals. The information for each hospital is arranged geographically within each section by town or city name and provides the name, address, and phone numbers for each institution, a code identifying its ownership and operating body, the licensure, and the year it was established. Brief statistics, number of beds and bassinets, personnel, and annual budget are provided to indicate level of activity. Chief administrators and department heads are also named.

Additional sections provide information on outpatient health services, poison control centers, provincial hospitals and health associations, educational programs for health personnel, associations of Canadian teaching hospital members, hospital construction, and hospital associations and allied organizations. A Buyers Guide provides information on hospital equipment and supplies. This section also has an index to advertisers by product and service, a listing of advertisers and distributors, and a general advertising index.

EDUCATION DIRECTORIES

13.31　*Admission Requirements of U.S. and Canadian Dental Schools.* Chicago, IL, American Association of Dental Schools. Vol. 1– , 1964/65– . Annual.

13.32　*State Approved Schools of Nursing—R.N., Meeting Minimum Requirements Set by Law and Board Rules in the Various Jurisdictions.* New York, NY, National League for Nursing. 25th ed. 1967– . (Continues *State-approved Schools of Professional Nursing.*) Annual.

13.33 *Medical School Admission Requirements, United States and Canada.* Washington, DC, Association of American Medical Colleges, 1951– . (Former title: *Admission Requirements of American Medical Colleges, Including Canada, 1951–1964/65.*) Annual.

13.34 *AAMC Directory of American Medical Education.* Washington, DC, Association of American Medical Colleges, 1967– . Annual.

Admission Requirements of U.S. and Canadian Dental Schools lists information for the fifty-nine United States, one Puerto Rican, and ten Canadian dental schools. Introductory chapters on "Dentistry as a Career" and "Planning a Dental Education" are followed by a geographic directory, arranged by states, territory, and provinces, as appropriate. Within the geographic arrangement, schools are listed alphabetically.

For each school, information is given on the basic program, admission requirements, selection factors, an admission timetable for the next class, financial aid, and estimated costs for four years. In addition, the characteristics of the most recent entering class are given, and names and addresses for further information on admission, housing, financial aid, and, for some schools, minority affairs are provided.

State Approved Schools of Nursing—R.N. is also a geographic listing. However, the information is presented in tabular form with abbreviations and codes. In all, 1,352 schools are listed for programs leading to the R.N. diploma, associate degree, or baccalaureate degree in the United States and territories. Alphabetically listed under each state are the name of the school, chairman or director of the program, address, type of program, National League for Nursing (NLN) accreditation status, administrative control, latest enrollment, admissions, and number of graduates. Summary tables are given for the number of programs, admissions, etc., by state. A directory of boards of nursing for the states and territories, as well as an alphabetical index by name of school, complete the volume. The NLN also publishes a number of other directories on nursing education and individual directories on the three R.N. programs, as well as licensed vocational nursing (LVN) and graduate programs.

Medical School Admission Requirements, too, presents a geographical arrangement of listings. Included are member schools of the Association of American Medical Colleges (AAMC). The information for each school in the United States and Puerto Rico, American University of Beirut, and Canada is presented in a similar format to that of the dental directory. Brief descriptions of the curricula, requirements for entrance, selection factors, financial aid, and information for minorities are followed by a timetable for application, estimated expenses for a year, and information on the latest entering class. Ten introductory chapters discuss such topics as the New Medical College Admissions Test (new MCAT), the nature of medical education, and information for applicants not admitted to medical school who are interested in pursuing a medical career outside the United States.

Complementing *Medical School Admission Requirements* is the *AAMC Directory of American Medical Education*. The bulk of the directory is a geographical listing of the schools. For each school the following information is provided: name, address, type of institution (public or private), total enrollment, clinical facilities, university officials, medical school administrative staff, and department and division section chairmen. Other sections of the *Directory* provide information on the AAMC organizational structure and activities, Council of Deans, Council of Academic Societies, Council of Teaching Hospitals, Organization of Student Representatives, and other members. An index to individuals mentioned in all of the sections of the *Directory* is also included.

13.35 *World Directory of Medical Schools 1979.* Geneva, World Health Organization, 1979.

13.36 Marion, Daniel. *Guide to Foreign Medical Schools.* New York, NY, Queens College Press/Institute of International Education, 1975.

13.37 Modica, Charles R. *Foreign Medical School Catalogue.* Bay Shore, NY, Foreign Medical School Information Center, 1971— . Annual.

The *World Directory of Medical Schools* is in its fifth edition. The information, based on a questionnaire sent to governments and individual schools, is arranged by country. The *Directory* is arranged by country, providing names and addresses of each school. Other pertinent information includes the date instruction began, admission requirements, length of medical studies, degrees awarded, language of instruction, and number of students admitted and graduated in 1976. Information is presented in English and French. "Annex," an appendix, lists each country, with the page in the directory where listings begin for that country, the number of medical schools in each country, and the country's population. In addition to the *World Directory of Medical Schools,* the World Health Organization publishes directories for other health schools, including veterinarians, animal health assistants, dentists, dental auxiliaries, and postbasic and postgraduate nursing.

The *Guide to Foreign Medical Schools* provides information for United States citizens seeking admissions to foreign medical schools, based on answers from questionnaires sent by the Institute of International Education to the various schools. The *Guide* is arranged geographically by country. Information varies for each country and institution depending on how thoroughly the questionnaires were answered. The *Guide* entries are written in a straightforward manner and will indicate if foreign (United States) students are accepted, whether there is a great deal of red tape, etc. A final chapter concerns returning to the United States after graduation with information on Educational Commission for Foreign Medical Graduates (ECFMG), the Coordinated Transfer Application System (COTRANS), and the Fifth Pathway program.

Both the above directories are referenced in *Medical School Admissions Requirements* for those individuals not admitted to United States medical schools who are still interested in pursuing a medical education.

More up-to-date information on foreign medical schools is available in Modica's *Foreign Medical School Catalogue,* which appears annually. Also arranged geographically, descriptive information on medical education in each country is followed by information about the schools, including administration (public or private), admission requirements, number of admissions, and graduates. Also provided are statistics on the ECFMG exam. These include the number taking the exam, the percent who pass, and the number of United States citizens who take and pass the exam. Introductory material provides general information on both ECFMG and COTRANS.

13.38 *Directory of Residency Training Programs Accredited by the Liaison Committee on Graduate Medical Education.* Chicago, IL, American Medical Association, 1978/79– . (Continues *Directory of Accredited Residencies.*) Annual.

13.39 *Directory of Clinical Fellowships in Medicine 1978–79 United States and Canada.* Ventura, CA, Graduate Publications, 1978.

The *Directory of Residency Training Programs* is much more than its title indicates. The bulk of the *Directory* is arranged by medical specialty, then geographically by state and city, then by institution. Included in this listing are the chief of the service or program director, statistical information about that service, and the number of available positions. In addition, introductory chapters provide information on graduate medical education, specialty studies, special reports, and a consolidated list of hospitals and medical school affiliations. There are also chapters on such topics as the National Intern and Resident Matching Program (NIRMP) and the Essentials of Accredited Residencies.

The *Directory of Clinical Fellowships in Medicine* in this first edition provides information on postresidency educational programs in medical subspecialties. Unlike the *Directory of Residency Training Programs,* where professional accreditation is required for inclusion, this directory lists both accredited and nonaccredited fellowships. It is divided into three sections: the first presents an analysis of fellowship training in the United States and Canada; the second section provides a geographically arranged list of medical centers with the types of fellowship programs they offer; and the third section lists the programs themselves. This last section is arranged by specialty, then geographically, and includes such information as the program director, cases seen per month, research available, number of starting positions, length of program, starting date, and stipend. Altogether, more than 1,200 programs are described.

The biographical sources and directories listed above are only a few of the vast number available. In the United States, regions, states, countries, and cities often issue directories of physicians, other health personnel, services, and organizations for their areas. A library should maintain directories of these local resources first, for a great number of its directory questions will undoubtedly be for local people and places. Again, the telephone directory can be an invaluable resource, and a library should maintain current phone books for its immediate and surrounding communities.

CHAPTER 14

History
Sources

SANDRA COLVILLE-STEWART

The focus here is not on rare, or older, medical works themselves, with the problems of their selection and acquisition, cataloging and preservation, but rather on the tools used to identify and provide further information about such works and their authors. It is fair to say that most medical reference librarians have to deal at some time with historical questions, even when their libraries have no historical or rare book collection. Indeed, there is a sense in which any book may be regarded as an historical reference tool. This is particularly true now, in view of the increasing interest in nineteenth- and twentieth-century medical history and in historical processes as well as personalities in medicine. In addition to their role as a complement to historical collections, such tools may also be of importance in other library functions: identifying possibly valuable works, receiving gifts, weeding collections, cataloging, or preparing exhibits.

14.1 Blake, John B., and Roos, Charles, eds. *Medical Reference Works, 1679–1966; A Selected Bibliography.* Chicago, IL, Medical Library Association, 1967. 3 supplements, 1970–75.

14.2 Smit, Pieter. *History of the Life Sciences: An Annotated Bibliography.* New York, NY, Hafner, 1974.

The following, necessarily brief, discussion is designed to give some indication of the types of materials available to answer the most common historical reference questions. The list is very highly selective, with all the inadequacies that follow. In every section there are available many additional tools—more specialized in their period, geographical or subject coverage, or even in other languages—so this discussion is also intended as a stimulus to lateral thinking. Most of the sources are listed in *Medical Reference Works, 1679–1966,* and supplements, which give more precise details as to their format and content, and also in the excellently annotated *History of the Life Sciences.* Although many of the sources described are now out of print, others are being reprinted or appear regularly on the secondhand market. A library that is serious about developing its historical reference collection should be able with patience to obtain most of the essential tools.

Most historical reference questions from library users fall into some six categories:

1. The identification, definition, and discovery of the source of medical eponyms, words, and phrases, particularly in Latin, which are found in the literature but are sometimes not included in standard medical dictionaries.
2. Information as to the properties of certain medicines or traditional herbal remedies.
3. Biographical information, perhaps the most common type of question to appear. The degree of difficulty in answering such queries depends upon the past importance of the individuals involved, their specialties, historical periods, and countries of origin.
4. Bibliographic information, such as the identification of incomplete or incorrect references, or of different editions of specific books; the location of copies of scarce works; the preparation of bibliographies by or about individuals, or about particular subjects.
5. Historical information about, for example: some specific disease or group of diseases; certain therapeutic methods, folk medicine, and quackery; particular medical institutions; the role of women in medicine; medical education and ethics; medicine as practiced in some particular place and time; the history of public health measures, of occupational medicine, of dentistry or nursing; the relationships between medicine and art, literature, or religion.
6. A need for pictorial representations of historical individuals or past medical events.

DICTIONARIES AND ENCYCLOPEDIAS

Dictionaries

14.3 James, Robert. *A Medicinal Dictionary* . . . London, T. Osborne, 1743–45. 3 vols.

14.4 Copland, James. *A Dictionary of Practical Medicine.* London, Longmans, etc. 1832–58. 3 vols.

14.5 *The New Sydenham Society's Lexicon of Medicine and the Allied Sciences.* London, The New Sydenham Society, 1881–99. 5 vols.

14.6 Clark, Paul F., and Clark, Alice S. *Memorable Days in Medicine.* Madison, WI, University of Wisconsin Press, 1942.

14.7 Strauss, Maurice B., ed. *Familiar Medical Quotations.* Boston, MA, Little, Brown, 1968.

The identification and definition of medical terms and phrases can often be achieved by means of the scientific and medical dictionaries in various languages to be found in standard medical reference collections, and no other reference sources have their information in such a condensed and economical form. Ideally, there should also be a chronological spread to such dictionaries to meet the historical need. Not only do terms disappear, but those that survive also change their meanings. Many such questions can also be answered from sources in some of the other categories to be described.

Medical dictionaries are found in the fifteenth century, but they became prominent as aids to knowledge in the eighteenth century. The *Medicinal Dictionary* of Robert James was the largest and most scholarly in English until the nineteenth century, when others, such as Copland's *A Dictionary of Practical Medicine* and the New Sydenham Society's *Lexicon of Medicine and the Allied Sciences,* appeared. The latter approaches the format of an encyclopedia, with long accounts of certain medical specialties. Some more modern dictionaries have been published with specifically historical intent, sometimes being limited to particular periods of medicine or the medical sciences in specific countries. Two examples of these very special forms are included here: a chronology or list of important dates in medicine, such as the dates of birth and death of important individuals or dates of important events; and a dictionary of quotations. There are several examples of chronologies, some listing events by year and others by day of the year, as in the Clarks' *Memorable Days in Medicine.* Such works are of especial importance, for example, in the planning of possible exhibits. The second, *Familiar Medical Quotations*, is just one example of several dictionaries of quotations with especial reference to medicine.

Encyclopedias

14.8 *Encyclopädisches Wörterbuch der medicinischen Wissenschaft.* Berlin, J. W. Boike, 1828–49. 37 vols.

14.9 *Dictionnaire encyclopédique des sciences médicales.* Paris, P. Asselin, etc., 1864–89. 100 vols.

The encyclopedias listed here are just two of several such magnificent multivolume works published in the nineteenth century. The second is of particular interest since it includes articles by some of the most prominent physicians of the time and has excellent bibliographies. Such texts now act as both primary and secondary sources of information. Unfortunately, they are now all of limited availability, but some of the more modern medical encyclopedias also include historical material, even if not of such fine quality.

Pharmacopeias

14.10 Gerard, John. *The Herbal: Or, General History of Plants*. The complete 1633 edition as revised and enlarged by Thomas Johnson. New York, Dover, 1975. (Facsimile)

Questions as to the ingredients and properties of historical medicines or herbal remedies, or the medical properties of certain plants, may often be answered using some of the tools to be described in later categories as well as from books in the regular library collections. Such works include older editions of the national pharmacopeias, listing of unofficial drugs, older works on pharmacology, and books on domestic medicine and therapeutics. There are available at present many excellent reprints and facsimiles of important medical works including some, although not enough, of the reference works discussed here. One such is the recent facsimile edition of Gerard's *Herbal*, valuable not only for its beauty and botanical information, but also for its usefulness as a reference tool in historical pharmacological questions. Other important early herbals are similarly available.

Biographical Dictionaries

GENERAL

14.11 Hirsch, August, ed. *Biographisches Lexikon der hervorragenden Aerzte aller Zeiten und Völker.* 2d ed. Berlin, Urban & Schwarzenberg, 1929–35. Reprint: München, Urban & Schwarzenberg, 1962. 5 vols. and supplement.

14.12 Fischer, I., ed. *Biographisches Lexikon der hervorragenden Aerzte der letzten fünfzig Jahre.* Berlin, Urban & Schwarzenberg, 1932–33. Reprint: München, Urban & Schwarzenberg, 1962. 2 vols.

14.13 Gillispie, Charles G., ed. *Dictionary of Scientific Biography.* New York, NY, Charles Scribner's Sons, 1970–76. 14 vols. and supplement.

14.14 Debus, Allen G., ed. *World Who's Who in Science. A Biographical Dictionary of Notable Scientists From Antiquity To The Present.* Chicago, IL, Marquis, 1968.

14.15 Talbott, John H., ed. *A Biographical History of Medicine.* New York, NY, Grune & Stratton, 1970.

14.16 New York Academy of Medicine Library. *Catalog of Biographies.* Boston, MA, Hall, 1960.

There are numerous specialized biographical dictionaries devoted to the medical and allied sciences, but information about many individuals of interest in these sciences may also be found in encyclopedias, national biographies, and in individual biographies, as well as in the bibliographic and historical tools here described. Moreover, a search begun in collective biographical dictionaries may well have to be extended for further details about an individual, and ideally this extension should be possible using bibliographic information gleaned from these works. The best biographical references, besides giving full names, dates of birth and death, life histories, particular medical advances, prominent associates, and places of work, go on to give a bibliography of the most important references by and about the individuals in question and also include a portrait, one of the most pressing needs of many patrons.

The most important biographical dictionaries specifically devoted to medicine, although by no means the earliest, are those by Hirsch and Fischer, which cover the period to 1930, the *Biographisches Lexikon der hervorragenden Aerzte aller Zeiten und Völker,* and the *Biographisches Lexikon der hervorragenden Aerzte der letzten fünfzig Jahre.* Although Hirsch contains few portraits and is in German (an English translation is projected), this tool has yet to be superseded by more recent sources.

One of the latest, and most useful, biographical dictionaries, the *Dictionary of Scientific Biography,* is especially valuable for the authoritative nature of the biographies and the lists of primary and secondary sources included. Although many medical figures of importance were unfortunately omitted, others can be found, because their work was of a more general scientific nature. Other sources of more concise biographical information include the *World Who's Who in Science. A Biographical Dictionary of Notable Scientists From Antiquity To The Present,* which is one of the few to include living scientists, and John H. Talbott's *A Biographical History of Medicine,* prepared chiefly from historical editorials in *Journal of the American Medical Association (JAMA).* The New York Academy of Medicine Library's *Catalog of Biographies* provides direct information, such as dates, in addition to the lists of biographical material that form the main part of the catalog.

SPECIFIC

14.17　Kelly, Howard A., ed. *A Cyclopedia of American Medical Biography . . . from 1610 to 1910.* Philadelphia, PA, Saunders, 1912. 2 vols.

14.18　Kelly, Howard A., and Burrage, Walter L. *American Medical Biographies.* Baltimore, MD, Norman, Remington, 1920.

14.19　Kelly, Howard A., and Burrage, Walter L. *Dictionary of American Medical Biography . . .* New York, NY, Appleton, 1928.

14.20　Royal College of Physicians of London. *Munk's Roll.* London, The College, 1878–1968. 5 vols.

14.21　Plarr, Victor G. *Plarr's Lives of the Fellows of the Royal College of Surgeons of England.* Revised by Sir D'Arcy Power. London, Simpkin, Marshall, 1930. 2 vols.

14.22　Talbot, Charles H., and Hammond, E. A. *The Medical Practitioners in Medieval England; A Biographical Register.* London, Wellcome Historical Medical Library, 1965.

14.23　Dezeimeris, Jean E. *Dictionnaire Historique de la Médecine, Ancienne et Moderne.* Paris, Béchet, 1838–39. 4 vols.

14.24 Haymaker, Webb, and Schiller, Francis, eds. *The Founders of Neurology* . . . 2d ed. Springfield, IL, Thomas, 1970.

14.25 Zusne, Leonard, ed. *Names in the History of Psychology: A Biographical Source Book.* Washington, DC, Hemisphere, 1975.

14.26 Gilbert, Judson B. *Disease and Destiny; A Bibliography of Medical References to the Famous.* London, Dawsons, 1962.

Other biographical dictionaries are more limited in scope, usually being devoted to individuals of specific countries, time periods, or subject specialties. Many give information only about United States physicians, some being further limited, for example, to the doctors of individual states or to those physicians involved in the American Revolution. The most valuable sources for information on American doctors are the three editions of Kelly's *Cyclopedia,* which have brief bibliographies but which may need to be supplemented by other sources. The contents of the three editions are only partially cumulative.

In a parallel manner there are two basic tools for the investigation of English physicians and surgeons: the biographical directory of the Royal College of Physicians of London, *Munk's Roll,* and *Plarr's Lives of the Royal College of Surgeons of England.* Again, other more specialized sources also exist, such as Talbot and Hammond's *The Medical Practitioners in Medieval England.* Similar tools are available specific to other European nations, one early example being the *Dictionnaire Historique de la Médecine, Ancienne et Moderne,* particularly useful because it is not confined to French practitioners.

Just as there are biographical dictionaries devoted to physicians of specific countries, so there are dictionaries for particular specialties and subject areas. Some of the most distinguished examples include Haymaker and Schiller's *The Founders of Neurology* and Zusne's *Names in the History of Psychology.*

One very common type of biographical reference question within the historical area concerns the medical history of famous individuals. Such questions are usually most fully answered by encyclopedias and specific biographies, but a very helpful general introductory tool is Gilbert's *Disease and Destiny; A Bibliography of Medical References to the Famous,* which, like other similar works, gives a brief bibliography for each individual, from Napoleon Bonaparte to Nebuchadnezzar.

BIBLIOGRAPHIES

The bibliographic tools of most importance in medical historical reference work, those that are used for finding secondary materials as well as for the verification and identification of original works, can be divided into three groups: (1) bibliographies of secondary materials; (2) general bibliographic indexes; (3) printed catalogs of collections.

1. Bibliographies of secondary materials, namely monographs and periodical articles devoted to the history of medicine and the life sciences:

14.27 *Current Work in the History of Medicine.* London, Wellcome Historical Medical Library. No. 1– , 1954– .

14.28 Whitrow, Magda, ed. *ISIS Cumulative Bibliography; A Bibliography of the History of Science Formed from ISIS Critical Bibliographies 1–90, 1913–65.* London, Mansell, in conjunction with the History of Science Society, 1971– . 3 vols.

14.29 *Bibliography of the History of Medicine.* Bethesda, MD, National Library of Medicine. No. 1– , 1965– . Cumulated every five years.

14.30 Miller, Genevieve, ed. *Bibliography of the History of Medicine of the United States and Canada, 1939–1960.* Baltimore, MD, Johns Hopkins Press, 1964.

14.31 Gilbert, Judson B., ed. *A Bibliography of Articles on the History of American Medicine, Compiled from "Writings on American History," 1902–1937.* New York, NY, New York Academy of Medicine, 1951.

14.32 Mann, Gunter, ed. *Internationale Bibliographie zur Geschichte der Medizin, 1875–1901.* New York, NY, Olms, 1970.

14.33 Watson, Robert I., ed. *Eminent Contributors to Psychology. Volume I. A Bibliography of Primary References. Volume II. A Bibliography of Secondary References.* New York, NY, Springer, 1974–76.

The fact that several such indexes exist is a reflection of the difficulty of controlling a literature that appears not only in a great diversity of formats but also in materials from many nonmedical disciplines. Three of the indexes are general, and essential: the quarterly *Current Work in the History of Medicine*; and the two annual and cumulated bibliographies, the *ISIS Cumulative Bibliography* and the *Bibliography of the History of Medicine.* All of these include books, journal articles, and often theses and exhibit catalogs as well. Each can be approached by subject, subdivided by historical period, as well as by author or biographical subject. The first two also include entries by institution and have a more specific subject breakdown. The Wellcome Historical Medical Library is now publishing its subject catalog, which also acts as the long-needed cumulation of the subject section of *Current Work in the History of Medicine.*

Some more limited national bibliographies also exist, for example, the *Bibliography of the History of Medicine of the United States and Canada, 1939–1960,* a supplement to *A Bibliography of Articles on the History of American Medicine . . . 1902–1937.* Others, like the *Internationale Bibliographie zur Geschichte der Medizin, 1875–1901,* cover only the earlier material or are of more limited subject scope, such as that by Pieter Smit (14.2) and Robert I. Watson's *Eminent Contributors to Psychology.*

2. General bibliographic indexes for the identification of primary and secondary medical materials of historical interest, both books and manuscripts:

14.34 *Index-Catalogue of the Library of the Surgeon General's Office* . . . Washington, DC, 1880–1961. 5 series.

14.35 Morton, Leslie T. *A Medical Bibliography (Garrison and Morton). An Annotated Check-list of Texts Illustrating the History of Medicine.* 3d ed. Philadelphia, PA, Lippincott, 1970.

14.36 Ash, Lee. *Serial Publications Containing Medical Classics; an Index to Citations in Garrison/Morton (3d ed., 1970).* 2d ed. Bethany, CT, Antiquarium 1979.

14.37 Choulant, Johann L. *Handbuch der Bücherkunde für die ältere Medizin* . . . 2d ed. Leipzig, Voss, 1841. Reprint: Graz, Akademische Druck, 1956.

14.38 Pauly, Alphonse. *Bibliographie des Sciences Médicales: Bibliographie—Biographie—Histoire—Épidémies—Topographies—Endémies.* Paris, Librarie Tross, 1874. Reprint: London, Verschoyle, 1954.

14.39 Kelly, Emerson C. *Encyclopedia of Medical Sources.* Baltimore, MD, Williams & Wilkins, 1948.

14.40 Jablonski, Stanley. *Illustrated Dictionary of Eponymic Syndromes and Diseases and Their Synonyms.* Philadelphia, PA, Saunders, 1969.

14.41   Austin, Robert B. *Early American Medical Imprints; A Guide to Works Printed in the United States, 1668–1820.* Washington, DC, Public Health Service, 1961.

14.42   Weinberger, Bernhard W., comp. *Dental Bibliography* . . . [pt. 1: *A Reference Index* . . . 2d ed.; pt. 2: *A Subject Index* . . .] New York, NY, First District Dental Society, 1929–32.

14.43   Thompson, Alice M. C., ed. *A Bibliography of Nursing Literature, 1859–1960.* London, Library Association, 1968. Supplement: London, 1974.

The most important of these general indexes is the *Index Catalogue of the Library of the Surgeon General's Office.* This index has a multiplicity of reference uses, from verification and the preparation of bibliographies by subject or author, to the supplying of biographical information and obituaries. It can indeed be described almost as an encyclopedia of biobibliography. Often the subject entries form histories in themselves. Other essential items in any historical reference collection are Morton's *A Medical Bibliography (Garrison and Morton)* and the supplementary publication compiled by Lee Ash, *Serial Publications Containing Medical Classics.* Devoted to medical "firsts," these two works are of prime importance in appraising the value of gifts for their historical importance and in historical collection development and weeding. Arranged by subject, Garrison and Morton is also of value in the preparation of exhibits.

Medicine has traditionally had an exceptionally good bibliography, and so many other general indexes are also available, dating back to the sixteenth century. Some of the more accessible, which are of particular value for their coverage of the early literature, include those by Johann L. Choulant, for example, the *Handbuch der Bücherkunde für die ältere Medizin,* and Alphonse Pauly's *Bibliographie des Sciences Médicales.* Other bibliographic tools in this category are especially useful to locate materials specific to certain eponymous syndromes and diseases. Examples include Kelly's *Encyclopedia of Medical Sources* and Jablonski's *Illustrated Dictionary of Eponymic Syndromes.*

There are also general bibliographic tools devoted to the literature of a particular country and/or period, for example, Austin's *Early American Medical Imprints:* to the literature of specific subject areas, such as plastic surgery, zoology, dentistry (*Dental Bibliography* edited by Weinberger), and nursing (Alice Thompson's *A Bibliography of Nursing Literature, 1859–1960*).

3. Bibliographies that are, for the most part, printed catalogs of important collections in the history of medicine, including both manuscripts and printed books and representing both general and specialized collections:

14.44 National Library of Medicine. *A Catalogue of Incunabula and Manuscripts in the Army Medical Library.* Compiled by Dorothy M. Schullian and Francis E. Sommer. New York, NY, Schuman, 1950. Supplement: Bethesda, MD, 1971.

14.45 ———. *A Catalogue of Sixteenth Century Printed Books in the National Library of Medicine.* Compiled by Richard J. Durling. Bethesda, MD, 1967. Supplement: Bethesda, MD, 1971.

14.46 Wellcome Historical Medical Library, London. *A Catalogue of Incunabula in the Wellcome Historical Medical Library.* Compiled by Frederick N. L. Poynter. London, Oxford University Press, 1954.

14.47 ———. *A Catalogue of Printed Books in the Wellcome Historical Medical Library.* London, Wellcome Historical Medical Library, 1962– . 2 vols.

14.48 Osler, Sir William, Bart. *Incunabula Medica: A Study of the Earliest Printed Medical Books, 1467–1480.* Oxford, Oxford University Press. 1923.

14.49 ———. *Bibliotheca Osleriana; A Catalogue of Books Illustrating the History of Medicine and Science.* Oxford, Clarendon Press, 1929. Reprint: Montreal, McGill-Queen's University Press, 1969.

14.50 John Crerar Library, Chicago. *Catalog of the Clifford G. Grulee Collection on Pediatrics.* Chicago, IL, 1959.

14.51 University of Reading. *The Cole Library of Early Medicine and Zoology: Catalogue of Books and Pamphlets.* Compiled by Nellie B. Eales. Oxford, Alden Press, 1969–75. 2 vols.

There is a very large number of such catalogs, useful primarily for identification and verification, and for the preparation of author or subject bibliographies. Some representative examples of the general type include catalogs from the National Library of Medicine, such as their *Catalogue of Incunabula and Manuscripts* and *Catalogue of Sixteenth Century Printed Books*; and from the Wellcome Historical Medical Library, London, which is one of the richest such collections in the world and which has published catalogues of several parts of the collection, including the *Catalogue of Incunabula* and the continuing *Catalogue of Printed Books*. There are also more personal catalogues representing the scholarship of Sir William Osler, which include the *Incunabula Medica* and the *Bibliotheca Osleriana*.

Catalogs of specialized collections, including those of medical societies such as the Royal College of Physicians of London and of universities, are obviously of great value for research in particular fields. They can be found in areas ranging from surgery and obstetrics to pediatrics (the *Catalog of the Clifford G. Grulee Collection on Pediatrics*) and zoology (the University of Reading's catalog of *The Cole Library of Early Medicine and Zoology*).

There also exist many bibliographies or biobibliographies devoted to specific famous medical personalities such as Florence Nightingale or Edward Jenner. Just as these bibliographies can give much biographical information, and vice versa, so can much biobibliography be achieved using general and special histories and source books of medicine and the allied sciences, some examples of which will be described in the following section.

HISTORIES AND SOURCE WORKS

Histories

GENERAL

14.52 Garrison, Fielding H. *An Introduction to the History of Medicine, with Medical Chronology, Suggestions for Study and Bibliographic Data*. 4th ed. Philadelphia, PA, Saunders, 1929.

14.53 Castiglioni, Arturo. *A History of Medicine*. Translated and edited by E. B. Krumbhaar. 2d ed. New York, NY, Knopf, 1947.

14.54 Major, Ralph H. *A History of Medicine*. Springfield, IL, Thomas, 1954. 2 vols.

14.55 Neuberger, Max. *History of Medicine*. Translated by E. Playfair. London, Frowde, 1910. 2 vols.

14.56 Sigerist, Henry E. *A History of Medicine*. New York, NY, Oxford University Press, 1951–61. 2 vols.

14.57 Entralgo, Pedro Laín, ed. *Historia Universal de la Medicina*. Barcelona, Salvat, 1972–75. 7 vols.

As may be imagined, there is an enormous number of histories that could be considered for inclusion here: encyclopedic histories that cover all periods and specialties, specific biographical studies and those devoted to single disease entities or institutions, histories of medical education or medical technology, and treatments of specialties as developed in particular countries, states, or periods. Many of the older works now show signs of age in their conceptual content, but they are still invaluable for biographical and bibliographic information and for their illustrations. Not perhaps the most immediately obvious of reference tools, such histories often best answer questions in the historical area. Those chosen here include some of the most specialized types merely as an indication of what is available.

Perhaps the most valuable reference history in English is still the encyclopedic work by Fielding H. Garrison, *An Introduction to the History of Medicine,* followed by that of Arturo Castiglioni. Other useful general histories include that by Ralph H. Major; the volumes by Henry E. Sigerist, the great medical historian; and Neuberger's *History of Medicine.* Finally, in this group should be included a multivolume Spanish work, the *Historia Universal de la Medicina,* that proves valuable not only for its wide scope, including contemporary medicine, but also for the lavish color and black-and-white illustrations.

SPECIFIC

14.58 Nordenskiöld, Erik. *The History of Biology; a Survey.* New York, NY, Tudor, 1949 (copyright 1928).

14.59 Singer, Charles J. *A History of Biology to about the Year 1900; a General Introduction to the Study of Living Things.* 3d ed. New York, NY, Abelard-Schuman, 1959.

14.60 Gardner, Eldon J. *History of Biology.* 3d ed. Minneapolis, MN, Burgess, 1972.

14.61 Nutting, Mary A., and Dock, Lavinia L. *A History of Nursing.* New York, NY, Putnam, 1907–12. Reprint: Buffalo, NY, Heritage Press, 1974. 4 vols.

14.62 Dolan, Josephine A. *Nursing in Society: A Historical Perspective.* 14th ed. Philadelphia, PA, Saunders, 1978.

14.63 Wangensteen, Owen H., and Wangensteen, Sarah D. *The Rise of Surgery from Empiric Craft to Scientific Discipline.* Minneapolis, MN, University of Minnesota Press, 1978.

14.64 Jetter, Dieter. *Geschichte des Hospitals*. Wiesbaden, Steiner, 1966–72. 3 vols.

14.65 Thompson, John D., and Goldin, Grace. *The Hospital: A Social and Architectural History*. New Haven, CT, Yale University Press, 1975.

14.66 Koch, Charles R. E., ed. *History of Dental Surgery*. Fort Wayne, IN, National Art, 1910. 3 vols.

14.67 Weinberger, Bernard W. *An Introduction to the History of Dentistry, with Medical & Dental Chronology & Bibliographic Data*. Vol. 2: *An Introduction to the History of Dentistry in America*. St. Louis, MO, Mosby, 1948. 2 vols.

14.68 Weinberger, Bernard W. *Orthodontics; an Historical Review of Its Origin and Evolution* . . . St. Louis, MO, Mosby, 1926. 2 vols.

14.69 Kremers, Edward. *Kremers' and Urdang's History of Pharmacy*. Revised by Glenn Sonnedecker. 4th ed. Philadelphia, PA, Lippincott, 1976.

14.70 Schelenz, Hermann. *Geschichte der Pharmazie*. Berlin, Springer, 1904. Reprint: Hildesheim, Olms, 1962.

Of the larger histories restricted to more limited subject or geographical areas, only a very few can be mentioned here, since each area usually has a multiplicity of specialized histories, biographical and bibliographic tools, and historical periodicals. Some important examples from biology, nursing, surgery, dentistry, and other allied sciences are included, however. There are several classic histories of biology such as those by Nordenskiold and Singer, followed by other more recent texts, for example, Gardner's *History of Biology*. Nursing is also represented by several substantial histories, some of the most authoritative being the early history by Nutting and Dock, *A History of Nursing*, and a regularly revised work, now by Dolan, *Nursing in Society: A Historical Perspective*. The recent history of surgery by the Wangensteens is full of useful information for the reference librarian.

Most histories of hospitals are limited to specific geographical areas or institutions. Nevertheless, there are a few general studies, for example, those of Jetter and of Thompson and Goldin. Dentistry and pharmacy are both better provided, with several excellent general histories. In dentistry the most substantial are Koch's *History of Dental Surgery* and those by Weinberger, which include *An Introduction to the History of Dentistry* and *Orthodontics*. For pharmacy *Kremers' and Ur-*

dang's History of Pharmacy and the earlier work by Hermann Schelenz, *Geschichte der Pharmazie,* are two of the most comprehensive and useful.

Source Works

14.71 Major, Ralph H., comp. *Classic Descriptions of Disease, with Biographical Sketches of the Authors.* 3d ed. Springfield, IL, Thomas, 1965.

14.72 Clendening, Logan, ed. *Source Book of Medical History.* New York, NY, Hoeber, 1942. Reprint: New York, NY, Dover, 1960.

14.73 Bloomfield, Arthur L. *A Bibliography of Internal Medicine: Selected Diseases.* Chicago, IL, University of Chicago Press, 1960.

14.74 ———. *A Bibliography of Internal Medicine: Communicable Diseases.* Chicago, IL, University of Chicago Press, 1958.

14.75 Long, Esmond R. *Selected Readings in Pathology.* 2d ed. Springfield, IL, Thomas, 1961.

14.76 Willius, Frederick A., and Keys, Thomas E., eds. *Classics of Cardiology.* New York, NY, Schuman, 1961. 2 vols.

14.77 Bick, Edgar M. *Source Book of Orthopaedics.* New ed. New York, NY, Hafner, 1968.

14.78 Speert, Harold. *Obstetric and Gynecologic Milestones; Essays in Eponymy.* New York, NY, Macmillan, 1958.

14.79 Fulton, John F., comp. *Selected Readings in the History of Physiology.* 2d ed. Springfield, IL, Thomas, 1966.

14.80 Clarke, Edwin, and O'Malley, Charles D. *The Human Brain and Spinal Cord; A Historical Study Illustrated by Writings from Antiquity to the Twentieth Century.* Berkeley, CA, University of California Press, 1968.

14.81 Holmstedt, Bo, and Liljestrand, G., eds. *Readings in Pharmacology.* New York, NY, Macmillan, 1963.

14.82 Austin, Anne L. *History of Nursing Source Book.* New York, NY, Putnam, 1957.

14.83 Hunter, Richard A., and MacAlpine, Ida. *Three Hundred Years of Psychiatry, 1535–1860; A History Presented in Selected English Texts.* London, Oxford University Press, 1963.

Within this section on histories, some mention should be made of source works in the history of medicine, namely those containing selected passages from original texts that were important contributions to knowledge. Usually these selections are devoted to particular groups of diseases and are accompanied by biographical and other historical information. Such tools are thus of value for the identification of valuable items as well as for answering the usual reference questions, but with a valuable extra dimension, that they include copies of the original texts. They are particularly popular with students and others beginning their work in the field, especially if the original works are not immediately available in the library.

Several of these anthologies attempt to cover most of the important discoveries in medicine, for example, those compiled by Ralph H. Major, *Classic Descriptions of Disease*, and by Logan Clendening, *Source Book of Medical History*. Most, however, are more limited in scope and devoted to some specialty, such as Bloomfield's two bibliographies of internal medicine; Long's *Selected Readings in Pathology*, Willius and Keys' *Classics of Cardiology*, and Bick's *Source Book of Orthopaedics*; and Harold Speert's *Obstetric and Gynecologic Milestones*. Some are restricted to specific facets of anatomy and physiology: the excellent *Selected Readings in the History of Physiology* by Fulton and Clark and O'Malley's authoritative *The Human Brain and Spinal Cord*. There are also many such tools in related areas such as pharmacy, nursing, dentistry, and psychiatry; some examples include Holmstedt and Liljestrand's *Readings in Pharmacology*, Austin's *History of Nursing Source Book*, and the invaluable *Three Hundred Years of Psychiatry*, 1535–1860, by Hunter and MacAlpine.

INDEXES TO ILLUSTRATIONS

GENERAL

14.84 Bettman, Otto L. *A Pictorial History of Medicine*. Springfield, IL, Thomas, 1956.

14.85 Laignel-Lavastine, Maxime, ed. *Histoire Générale de la Médécine, de la Pharmacie, de l'Art Dentaire et de l'Art Vétérinaire*. Paris, Michel, 1936–49. 3 vols.

14.86 Holländer, Eugen. *Die Medizin in der klassischen Malerei*. 4th ed. Stuttgart, Enke, 1950.

14.87 ———. *Die Karikatur und Satire in der Medizin*, 2d ed. Stuttgart, Enke, 1921.

14.88 ———. *Plastik und Medizin*. Stuttgart, Enke, 1912.

14.89 Herrlinger, Robert. *Geschichte der medizinischen Abbildung.* München, Moos, 1967–72. 2 vols.

14.90 Lyons, Albert S., and Petrucelli, R. Joseph. *Medicine: An Illustrated History.* New York, NY, Abrams, 1978.

14.91 Library of the New York Academy of Medicine. *Illustration Catalog.* 2d ed. Boston, MA, Hall, 1965.

14.92 ———. *Portrait Catalog.* Boston, MA, Hall, 1959– . 5 vols. and supplements.

14.93 Royal College of Physicians of London. *Portraits.* Edited by Gordon Wolstenholme. London, Churchill, 1964–77. 3 vols.

14.94 LeFanu, William R. *A Catalogue of the Portraits and Other Paintings, Drawings and Sculpture in the Royal College of Surgeons of England.* Edinburgh, Livingstone, 1960.

14.95 Wellcome Institute of the History of Medicine. *Portraits of Doctors & Scientists in the Wellcome Institute of the History of Medicine;* A Catalogue by Renate Burgess. London, 1973.

Many of the materials already mentioned, and many other comparable works in each category, are profusely illustrated. However, there are some tools of especial use when searching for visual material depictions of medical techniques, older anatomical and pathological illustrations, pictures of particular institutions, or portraits of individuals. Often the accompanying texts are excellent, supplying valuable historical details. Many are devoted to medicine in general, while others are particularly useful in the study of specific areas.

Among the general works giving illustrations must be included Laignel-Lavastine's excellent *Histoire Générale de la Médécine,* the three classic studies by Eugen Holländer, and *A Pictorial History of Medicine;* this last book is based on the contents of the Bettman Archive in New York City and is lavishly illustrated, although the reproduction and documentation are sometimes poor. Finally, there are Robert Herrlinger's *Geschichte der medizinischen Abbildung,* which is somewhat more accessible than most of the others because the first volume has also been published in English, and the more recent and lavish *Medicine: An Illustrated History* by Lyons and Petrucelli.

Although they themselves are not illustrated, two catalogs from the Library of the New York Academy of Medicine, the *Illustration Catalog* and the *Portrait Catalog,* act as indexes to thousands of sources of such visual materials. Portraits are always in demand, and other useful portrait catalogs include those from the collections of the Wellcome Institute of the History of Medicine.

Specific

14.96   Choulant, Johann L. *History and Bibliography of Anatomic Illustration.* New York, NY, Schuman, 1945. Reprint: New York, NY, Hafner, 1962.

14.97   Clarke, Edwin, and Dewhurst, Kenneth. *An Illustrated History of Brain Function.* Berkeley, CA, University of California Press, 1972.

14.98   Speert, Harold. *Iconographia Gyniatrica; A Pictorial History of Gynecology and Obstetrics.* Philadelphia, PA, Davis, 1973.

14.99   Roback, Abraham A., and Kiernan, Thomas, *Pictorial History of Psychology and Psychiatry.* New York, NY, Philosophical Library, 1969.

14.100 Proskauer, Curt. *Iconographia Odontologica.* 2d ed. Berlin, H. Meusser, 1926. Reprint: Hildesheim, Olms, 1967.

14.101 Proskauer, Curt, and Witt, Fritz H. *Bildgeschichte der Zahnheilkunde; Zeugnisse aus 5 Jahrtausenden.* Köln, Dumont Schauberg, 1962.

14.102 Bennion, Elisabeth. *Antique Medical Instruments.* Berkeley, CA, University of California Press, 1979.

14.103 Velter, André, and Lamothe, Marie-José. *Les Outils du Corps.* Paris, Hier et Demain, 1978.

Examples of a more specialized nature include the standard reference work by the great medical bibliographer Johann L. Choulant, *History and Bibliography of Anatomic Illustration;* Dewhurst's *An Illustrated History of Brain Function;* Speert's *Iconographia Gyniatrica;* and Kiernan's *Pictorial History of Psychology and Psychiatry.* There are also two classic studies of dental illustration by Proskauer, his *Iconographia Odontologica* and, with Witt, the *Bildgeschichte der Zahnheilkunde; Zeugnisse aus 5 Jahrtausenden.* . . . Finally, two recent books help to fill an urgent need for comprehensive illustrated histories of medical instruments, Bennion's *Antique Medical Instruments* and Velter and Lamothe's *Les Outils du Corps.*

For many of the tools mentioned above, there are probably at least ten others that are as adequate or could supply information not contained in those chosen. The very basic general biographical and bibliographical items are indeed unique, but so many reference questions in the historical field can be readily answered by consulting specialized histories and biographies that selection of the latter for such an outline as this can only be painfully arbitrary. There are several journals that specialize in medical history and are also useful in reference work. Sometimes questions can only be answered by consulting the original works, many of which are now available in excellent reprints, modern translations, and microfilm. HISTLINE (History of Medicine On-line), the data base available from the National Library of Medicine, which is prepared from their *Bibliography of the History of Medicine, Index Medicus, Current Catalog,* and additional selected journals and other related publications, must also be remembered. The reference needs of the users, the existing strengths of the library's holdings, the allocated budget, and, finally, the continuing availability of such materials must be the final arbiters of choice.

READINGS

Cavanagh, G. S. T. Rare Books, Archives, and the History of Medicine. In: Annan, Gertrude L., and Felter, Jacqueline, W. *Handbook of Medical Library Practice.* 3d ed. Chicago, IL, Medical Library Association, 1970. pp. 254–283.

Clarke, Edwin, ed. *Modern Methods in the History of Medicine.* London, University of London, Athlone Press, 1971.

Gaskell, E. Historical and biographical sources. In: Morton, L. T., ed. *Use of Medical Literature.* 2d ed. London, Butterworths, 1977. pp. 414–440.

Waserman, Barbara, and Waserman, Manfred. The History of Medicine. A Bookshelf for the Public Library. *Libr. J.* 97:37–41, Jan 1972.

INDEX

A

J

K

L

O

P